the Healing Compass

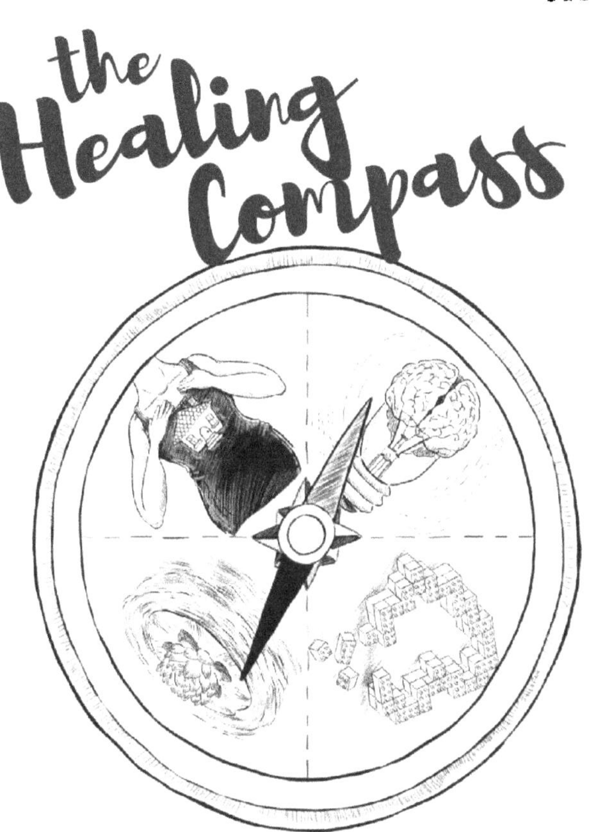

Find Your Roadmap to a Healthy, Happy Life

Angie Schickerowski

Illustrated by Amber Solberg

This book is not intended as a substitute for the medical advice of physicians. The reader should regularly consult a physician in matters relating to his/her health and particularly with respect to any symptoms that may require diagnosis or medical attention.

Cover Design & Illustrations: Amber Solberg
Book Illustrations: Amber Solberg
Edited By: Erin Dyrland
Author Photo: Lyndsay Greenwood

ISBN: 1985405423
ISBN-13: 978-1985405424

To the loves of my life
- Mike, Cassie, Lincoln & Savannah -
You are everything in the world to me.
Here's to a life full of more adventures:
Travelling the world,
Sundaes on Sunday,
Giggles and Dance Parties,
Bookapalooza's,
Camping and Exploring,
And Huggles every single day...

Contents

Start Now

"To live is the rarest feeling in the world.
Most people just exist."
~ Oscar Wilde ~

I felt stuck.

My wheels were turning, but I was getting nowhere - in so many different areas of my life.

I kept making the same goals over and over again, but I never made progress. I wanted to exercise more, but I never had the energy to even get started. I had a to-do list that was seven miles long, but more things were added than were ever crossed off.

I was busy and overwhelmed. I was exhausted and I felt alone, even when surrounded by amazing family and friends.

The most frustrating thing of all was that I was working so hard to become unstuck. I kept trying different things, consumed by the vision that I would find my path to health and happiness if I just kept trying.

That path shouldn't be so hard to navigate, right? Eat well, be active, always keep learning, build healthy relationships, and practice self-care. That sounds like an easy formula.

Except when life keeps handing you lemons.

You know what this is like. Maybe it's a health struggle - a diagnosis that leaves you blindsided or possibly a pile of symptoms that leave you and your doctor baffled. Maybe it's a major loss in your life - the death of a loved one, or a relationship breakup or breakdown. Maybe it's a stressful time you're going through - infertility, job loss or job insecurity, a child with special needs, or a cycle of self-doubt and self-sabotage.

We try to deal with those lemons while living in a world filled with disconnection, distractions, clutter, and chaos. That's the recipe for disaster. That's the perfect setup for getting stuck.

On the other hand, the recipe for getting unstuck sounds just as simple: **Heal your Body, Mind, Heart, & Soul.**

Let's face it - if it was that easy we would all be doing it. Meanwhile we're dodging lemons while knowing what *needs* to be done, but really lacking in the *how-to* department.

You see, these life events that cause imbalance (ex. illness, loss, or major stress), they don't come with a nice warning ahead of time, allowing us to prepare for their arrival. Cripes, they don't even ring the doorbell. They're the epitome of the overbearing, annoying houseguest that barges in unannounced and overstays their welcome.

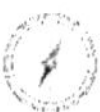

The first big lemon I received was a chronic health diagnosis in my early 20's.

It felt like I was spontaneously dropped off in a dense jungle with limited tools to find my way out. Every medication I tried took me to another dead end. Every alternative approach I explored seemed to give me one more tool for my belt, but never led me out of the jungle like I had hoped.

Then, the lemons kept showering down when we lost my dad to cancer and five years later suddenly lost my sister as well. With every major loss, my jungle became denser and the weather became incredibly unstable. Not only was I hacking my way through overgrown brush with a pair of dull scissors, but I was doing so in a torrential downpour.

At least that's what it felt like some days. One step forward was always met with two steps back. I kept trekking through that jungle, mapping my way as I went, but I kept hitting roadblocks and dead ends.

I couldn't get rid of this vision I had, of a healthy life full of purpose and passion. Where my husband, kids, and myself were travelling the globe. Where my soul was alive with the drive and determination to do big things and make a difference in the world. Where my successes became much greater than my struggles.

Over time, with the help of some wonderful mentors, I became more focused on taking care of myself. I finally understood that my illness, although physical in nature, could be better managed by spending time working on all areas of myself – my Body, Mind, Heart, and Soul. When I started intentionally working on healing myself, major shifts happened. My family noticed changes in my moods and energy. I saw improvements in the amount of pain and fatigue I was experiencing. My doctors' visits decreased substantially and test results showed tangible differences in my overall health.

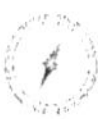

After twelve years of bushwhacking my way through the jungle, the path before me was becoming clear and I could finally see this beautiful horizon and scenery in front of me. Twelve years?! I felt as accomplished as Christopher Columbus sailing across the ocean and finding lands that have never been mapped before.

Wouldn't it be great if we were given a GPS or instruction manual to handle these situations? A set of personalized directions delivered by someone with an awesome Aussie accent? Or someone to hold our hand and give us encouraging support as we build our own personal roadmap to health and happiness?

The Healing Compass will do just that (minus the Aussie

accent). After learning how to assess your health in four areas - Body, Mind, Heart, and Soul - you will build good habits into your life to support and nourish those areas and your overall well-being. I'm here to help walk you through the entire process.

We're not talking earth-shattering life changes either. Read the table of contents - "Eat Like Great Grandma" or "Your Brain Needs Fuel Too". These are going to be simple shifts to your life. Chances are, you're already doing a few of them. But if you become very deliberate and intentional about how you make them a regular part of your life, that's when you'll see the magic happen.

You will become a better parent and partner, a better friend and colleague. Most importantly, you will become more in love with the amazing person that you are - your genuine self. The **you** that will be able to start living life to the fullest, and start making your dreams become reality.

Don't put it off until tomorrow because life happens. There's always something 'more important' on our to-do lists than taking care of ourselves. Always. Let's change that.

Start now.

A Very Large Nutshell

"It's important that we share our experiences with other people. Your story will heal you and your story will heal somebody else. When you tell your story, you free yourself and give other people permission to acknowledge their own story."
~ *Iyanla Vanzant* ~

What comes to mind when you hear somebody say, "to make a long story short..."? My mind jumps to the translation "get comfy, we're going to be here for a while...".

I would like to dive straight into the meat and potatoes of this book - helping you discover your path to health and happiness through using your Healing Compass. However, I feel I need to qualify myself as your guide first. To do that, I'll share my story with you, condensed into a nutshell. I just have to warn you that we're looking at a rather large nutshell, more like a coconut.

There are many parts of this story that used to bring about embarrassment and shame. Talking about bowel movements and how I permanently wear an ostomy bag (a device that holds my waste on the outside of my body), doesn't come naturally or easily.

However, along this journey I have found my voice and my courage. I am proud of my story and its scars. Those parts that I used to view as ugly and embarrassing - I now see as the pivotal parts of my journey that have made me who I am. They have been gifts to lead me to the place I am today.

That being said, this book isn't titled "Angie's Entire Medical History" for a reason. If you ever want to visit that novel, it sits in my doctor's filing cabinet - and it's really bulky, heavy, and difficult to piece together.

I became quite sick in the fall of 2004 with stomach aches, very irregular bowel movements, and the biggest 'OMG, something's wrong' indicator - bloody stools. Looking back, I was ill with other symptoms for about a year before that, but tummy troubles are so easy to be overlooked and brushed aside because often "it could just be something I ate...".

The city I lived in was in the middle of a boom and there were zero doctors taking on new patients, so my only option was to visit a walk-in clinic. That should have been no big deal. Yet, in the course of eight months I saw five different doctors and found myself in the middle of a misdiagnosis train wreck.

In October 2004, it was first labelled as food poisoning and I was instructed to eat bland foods and fill a prescription for antibiotics. When nothing improved I went back to the same clinic two weeks later where a different doctor diagnosed me with hemorrhoids and I was told to get an over the counter cream from the pharmacy. I suffered through another month of pain and bleeding, figuring that it would get better with time.

But things got worse, and before Christmas I returned to the same clinic. Part of me was hoping to see one of the same two doctors I had initially seen for consistency's sake. The other part of me was hoping it would be a brand new doctor who would know immediately what the issue was and how to heal me. I remember waiting for over two hours to be seen, hoping I would receive an early Christmas present in the form of a doctor delivering a correct diagnosis and proper treatment.

I think I was praying to the wrong God(s), because instead of a compassionate doctor with the gift of knowing the ins and outs of digestive issues, I was granted a condescending, over-tired physician who barely glanced at my file and told me that I likely had IBS (Irritable Bowel Syndrome). Her words and tone were straightforward and abrupt as she told me that I was making my symptoms ten times worse by drinking alcohol and eating an unhealthy diet. I felt ashamed, belittled, and terrible. She sent me off to do bloodwork and stool samples, and a month passed with me never hearing back from the doctor or the clinic.

I made some changes to my diet, but the truth was no matter what I ate, I was in so much pain. I started believing that I was the root cause of the symptoms I was experiencing. Instead of it becoming easier for me to talk about painful bowel movements, bloody stools, and ongoing diarrhea - I didn't want to discuss it at all. I didn't want to go back to another doctor. I knew deep down that something was very wrong with me, but my voice felt muted and I became discouraged.

More time went by, and at the end of January 2005 I finally went back to the clinic, armed with the intention of being assertive and expressing my concerns that something was seriously wrong and I needed further testing to figure it out. My assertiveness went out the window as my emotions bubbled over, and I was a sobbing mess as I tried to articulate what I was there for.

The doctor looked over my chart describing my previous visits, reviewed the bloodwork I had done, and with compassion in his voice told me that he wanted to refer me to a gastrointestinal specialist for further testing. "These symptoms have been going on far too long," he explained matter-of-factly. "You are also quite anemic and we should get you scheduled for an iron infusion right away."

That wasn't a surprise - I had been pooping blood every day for months on end.

I felt relieved and I was excited that my voice had finally been heard. Someone cared enough to send me to a doctor who specialized in the problems I was facing. As is often the case, the waitlist to see a specialist was quite long. An appointment was made for November, nine months later. I tried to hang on and wait.

My occupation at the time was a nanny, as I was in between two university degrees. It was a convenient occupation as I could often be very close to the bathroom for all of the troubles I had with my digestive system. One day while at work, the kids and I walked to a nearby park for a picnic lunch. After some playtime, we were on our way home and it was all I could do to get to the end of that last block, carting two kids and a backpack full of picnic supplies. We rushed into the house, I turned on cartoons for the kids and raced to the bathroom.

While I was in the bathroom, I curled up on the floor and I realized that I had hit a brick wall. I couldn't live like this anymore. The pain was intense, the blood clots leaving my body were huge, and the thought of waiting six more months made me cry.

My best friend Tracy took me to the emergency room and we waited over seven hours to be seen. Eventually, they told me that my bloodwork showed dehydration and anemia. I was given an iron infusion, IV hydration and was prepped for an emergency colonoscopy. I was introduced to the doctor that I still have to this day. He was a resident at that time, and his extremely knowledgeable yet caring demeanor was comforting from day one.

"You have ulcerative colitis," he told me after the colonoscopy, as he sat by my bedside, sharing more information and details. He sent me home with some corticosteroids (Prednisone), which would reduce my inflammation. The clinic would call to book me in for an immediate follow up to discuss medications and the next courses of action.

Ulcerative colitis (UC) is a form of Inflammatory Bowel Disease (IBD). It affects portions of the large intestine, including the rectum and anus, where inflammation and ulcers form in the intestinal lining. The symptoms are severe and can include bloody diarrhea, intense abdominal cramping, nausea, vomiting, false urges to have bowel movements, anemia, and fatigue.

Another part of UC that is important to understand is that it is also an autoimmune disorder. This means the immune system, which is normally designed to attack invading cells in the body, instead decides to haphazardly attack the healthy cells as well. In the case of UC, our T-cells attack the harmless, healthy bacteria of our large intestine causing inflammation and ulcers in the intestinal lining.

Now imagine the food we eat traveling over those open sores and ulcers in the large intestine. It's similar to having paper cuts on your hand and sticking it in a jar full of pickle juice. Ouch, right?

But back to my doctor's bedside visit. I heard the phrases "chronic disease" and "life-long condition" throughout my doctor's talk, but their weight didn't settle on my shoulders right away. Instead, I felt relief and comfort that I finally had an answer, and that the answer had steps to take towards helping me feel healthy again.

My first step after being released from the hospital was to hit up the local book store and stock pile books that would help me learn everything I could about this disease, the pros and cons of every medication, and what I could do to help heal myself.

I knew early on that a blend of modern medicine with alternative or complementary medicine was the route that I wanted to pursue. I understood the significance of a "forever" diagnosis, or at least thought I did. I imagined a lifetime of having these occasional disease flare-ups, but that overall I would lead a healthy life by managing my symptoms and getting every single flare-up under control.

My vision didn't exactly become reality. For three solid years I experienced a moderate flare-up every few months. I was diagnosed at 25 years old. Those years of being a 20-something with a disease that often left me tied to a toilet or even worse, not making it to the toilet, left lifelong scars on my emotional well-being.

That being said, I tried making lemonade every chance I had. I forced myself to see the bright side of everything. "At least I'm not dying," I would tell myself and push through the self-pity and sadness with a smile and a lame "This is shitty..." joke to try and make light of the whole situation.

Whenever my symptoms would start to ease up or disappear, I would get excited and declare myself in "remission", but the reality was that whatever medication I was on was working temporarily. Time and time again, within a few months the symptoms would reappear, my doctor would order another test or procedure, and a new medication would be prescribed.

Every single medication had unwelcome side effects. Whether it was weight gain, mood swings, headaches, nausea, or a weakened immune system, my overall health and wellness was on a constant roller coaster for many years.

Finding the courage to date somebody during those years of being full of disease was hard. Yet miraculously, I met my husband Mike in February 2007 in the middle of a bad flare-up. The first few months of dating were difficult as I would often cancel at last minute if I was having a bad day. When we did get together at his place for a movie date, I felt so embarrassed asking him to pause a movie three times so that I could run to the bathroom and have my insides explode into the toilet.

Mike was full of compassion and understanding, and thank goodness for his insistence on always communicating about every.little.thing, as it made those first few months together less stressful. When he shared his own medical challenges it became quite clear that our paths had crossed on purpose.

We spent our first Christmas together on a one week vacation to Cuba. We had an amazing time, but while I was there some disease symptoms began appearing. However, they could have easily been caused by a food or travel bug, so I didn't pay much attention to them.

After getting home, we celebrated New Year's Eve at a friend's house and I spent half the night traveling back and forth to the bathroom. I could tell something was wrong, and in the two weeks following that night, the train went seriously off the rails.

By the time I was able to see my GI doctor in mid-January 2008, I was having 28 bowel movements a day and losing blood clots the size of golf balls. Over the three years prior to this, I went through the gamut of prescriptions available for IBD, but none had worked very well. So, I was given the option of a clinical drug trial. It sounded like the perfect fit for me, given that the only other option would be surgery and at that time the prospect of surgery and living with a permanent ostomy was not something I was willing to consider.

The paperwork, red tape, and testing involved to get started on a clinical drug trial was intense. After signing a 49 page contract, and passing every test that needed to happen, I started the process of sticking a needle into my tummy once a week. I was also required to meet my nurses at the clinic every two weeks for bloodwork and to make sure everything was going okay.

Looking back, there were many aspects of that drug trial and the potential side effects that should have scared the bejeebers out of me. Yet, I held on to so much hope and faith that this was going to be the golden elixir. The one magical thing that would make me healthy again.

Two months into that trial, in April 2008, Mike proposed to me. We spent most of that spring and summer doing as much camping in our new-to-us motorhome as we possibly could. It turned out to be the best thing for us as it was a bathroom on wheels. We spent our weekends out of the city, doing something we loved to do and I remained close to a bathroom at all times. It doesn't get much better than that.

At the same time, throughout that entire spring and summer, my health continued to fail me. My focus on being a master lemonade maker stayed strong and I celebrated the fact that my bowel movements had reduced from 28 to 9 per day. I was delusional enough to convince myself that 9 trips to the bathroom to have my insides explode into the toilet, was a completely acceptable 'normal'.

In September of that year, I hit a point where I was having trouble walking. The inflammation was pushing on nerves in my lower spine and it hurt so bad to move. At the next visit with my research nurses, my angel of a nurse Val told me that she felt I needed to get off of the drug trial. "There are other options Angie," she told me with a hug, "You deserve better than this."

"Other options?" I thought, "Wasn't this the last medical option available?" Oh… right. That whole surgery conversation. An expedited visit with my GI doctor in late September told me the same thing. I finished the same paperwork and red-tape to get out of the drug trial, as it was obviously not working and my last and final option was to have surgery to remove my large intestine and live with either a J-pouch or a permanent ostomy. An appointment was made for six weeks later with a surgeon to discuss options.

In the meantime, high doses of prednisone were prescribed to try and get the inflammation under control. I lucked out with some of the prednisone side effects. My "moon face" (literally your face rounds out like a moon, complete with the marks and all) was minimal, and depression never took hold. However the manic side did. Who scrubs the crisper drawers of a fridge at 6:00 a.m.? This girl. Who creates a wedding cake topper out of modelling clay at midnight when her fiancé is away for one night? This girl.

Three weeks passed and I was hitting rock bottom.

I didn't actually realize it at the time. I was pushing through the best that I could, but Mike was worried about me every day and my best friend Jen said that I looked like I was on Death's doorstep. At a follow-up visit with my specialist, I was told to get myself admitted through emergency and I would have the surgery ASAP. There was no time to wait for the actual surgeon consult.

Until this point, I didn't actually believe I would be having surgery. I had an appointment with a surgeon, but that was just to discuss possible approaches. This new plan scared the shit out of me. I got in touch with everyone I knew through the power of Facebook and suddenly I had 100 close friends and family in my corner. All of the people that I knew I could always turn too, yet I never had... and they were there in a heartbeat offering support in whatever way they could.

Jen drove Mike and myself to the hospital where I was admitted. When the admitting nurse asked what my pain level was and I answered "about a 6 out of 10...", Jen flew off the handle in the most loving way possible.

"You are not Superwoman. You DO NOT need to BE Superwoman. Tell her what your pain is..." Jen said to me through gritted teeth, but still with an immense amount of love and compassion in her voice.

"It's a nine or nine-and-a-half..." I sobbed.

Needless to say, they got me on pain meds right away, which were a godsend as I waited an additional three days for surgery. Although I was admitted through emergency, they still had to attend to regularly scheduled surgeries and traumas above me. At one point I shared a room with three other patients including one obnoxious fellow who happened to be shot in the leg during a drug deal gone bad. Mike lost his mind on the surgical staff over the fact that this idiot might bump me out of surgical position. It turned out his insanely disrespectful behaviour to every single staff member did not work in his favour and I did get into the surgical room ahead of him.

There were two amazing women who changed the course of my history during that pre-surgery hospital stay. Two women who also had ostomy surgery in their younger years, and were dedicated to showing patients how fulfilling their lives could be living with an ostomy. Sheri and Lisa gave me so much hope with their openness and compassion. Combined with the incredible support of friends and family, this helped me see from day one that this surgery was saving my life and for that, I would be forever grateful.

My ostomy surgery involved a total colectomy which means the surgeon removed the entire large intestine. Then he created a stoma by pulling part of the small intestine through an opening he created on my abdomen. This stoma is where all of my waste leaves my body, and empties into an ostomy bag, which is an adhesive bag that attaches to the skin around my stoma. I have to empty the bag throughout the day as it fills with waste, and I change the entire pouching system roughly twice a week.

I was ready to move on to the healthy life that I had always envisioned and a permanent ostomy bag wasn't going to change that. My surgeon did a beautiful job on the surgery, but his surgical team made one major mistake. They kept talking about how this surgery would cure me. Without a colon, there is no more colitis. I believed I was cured and I could only imagine a life full of health and happiness ahead of me.

Recovery from the surgery was difficult, but it was also

amazing not to have the same pain as before. Adapting to life with an ostomy was relatively easy for me, and having a supportive partner helped immensely. It also helped having friends like Shireen who took me out shopping for some new wardrobe items, insisting we could find things that flattered my shape and hid the ostomy bag. And we did! A few months later she surprised me by taking me out to brunch with a "quick stop" at a wedding dress store, just to try some on for fun. Three dresses in and we found "the one". She knew exactly what I needed to help my confidence, and I am so grateful for that.

Mike and I were married in September 2009, ten months after my surgery. It was everything I ever hoped it would be. That December we spent almost three weeks in Cancun, Mexico on what we called our mini-moon. It was a trial run for an adventure we would soon set out on. Despite a bout of food poisoning that landed me in the hospital in Phoenix on our way home, the trial run was a success!

In May 2010, we left on a seven month journey travelling to Mexico, Belize, Honduras, Nicaragua, Costa Rica, Panama, and Peru. We flew back home to spend some time with family that summer and then we were back on the road exploring China, Vietnam, Cambodia, Thailand, Malaysia, Singapore, and Hong Kong. We called this adventure our Full Moon and it was the trip of a lifetime, brought to life by many months of saving, planning, and having faith while taking a giant leap outside of our comfort zones.

Traveling with an ostomy came with its challenges, especially the extensive travels we were doing. We carried extra supplies with us at all times, split amongst our backpacks and carry-ons so that if we ever lost luggage, I would still be covered. My best friend back home was equipped with extra stashes of my supplies and prepared to courier them to us anywhere in the world should it ever come to that. We researched medical centers and hospitals ahead of time and Mike plotted them in the GPS that we brought with us. We travelled through multiple airports, each security screening unique because I can't control when my ostomy bag fills up. Sometimes it chose to balloon from my abdomen at inopportune times like right before going through airport security. An officer in China poked at my bag once, asking what it was (in Mandarin of course) and I said "medical" repeatedly while my husband reached for a piece of paper that described the ostomy in 26 languages with pictures. She waved me through, no harm done. I've explained my ostomy to countless airport security personnel, occasionally going through full body scans, swabs, and pat downs. Every single time I choose to feel empowered that I can help educate them on something they may know little about.

Returning from such extensive travels left me feeling that absolutely nothing could stop me from achieving any dream or goal I had. Except for these potholes in the road that kept slowing me down. My health was far from perfect. I often tried to pretend that everything was great, but I had abdominal pain, my joints were often inflamed and sore, and even though my intestine was no longer attached to my rear end, the small amount of rectum that had been left behind leaked blood and mucus on a regular basis.

The surgeon had left behind what's called a rectal stump on purpose, because the surgery involved to remove it had high infertility risks associated with it. He knew we planned on starting our family within the next few years and suggested that we hold off until we had our babies, and then have a follow-up surgery.

We took our family planning seriously and in the span of two and a half years our family grew from two to five. Shortly after returning from our Full Moon, we decided to become foster parents to an incredible little five year old girl we knew needed a forever home. The road to adoption was a long one, but worth every struggle along the way. Mixed in with the fostering and adopting process, we had two healthy pregnancies, with our son born in September 2011, and our second daughter in April 2013.

In this same timeframe, we lost my dad to cancer. He was diagnosed in June 2011 when I was six months pregnant, and passed away five months later. I had a newborn and we were navigating the challenging road of helping our little girl who had been through so much trauma the first five years of her life. I never properly grieved the loss of my dad, and I have no doubt that the big ball of grief I carried around for years contributed to the health struggles I was facing.

My health continued on the roller coaster ride, and shortly after our youngest was born we decided that our family was complete at five. I booked the consult with my surgeon and when our baby was 10 months old I had my second major surgery to remove my diseased rectum. In the ostomy community we refer to this as Barbie Butt surgery, because our rear ends are sewn shut forever.

Recovery had its challenges again, but I was happy to be rid of more of the disease. However, I wasn't cured.

The next two years saw me go through many different struggles. I kept experiencing abdominal pain that x-rays and CT scans couldn't identify as anything other than a buildup of scar tissue from surgery and years of disease. I was experiencing chronic fatigue and attempting to just be a mom and wife was a struggle. I carefully planned my daily tasks to make sure I wouldn't physically over exert myself, as the simple act of showering could do me in.

Then, I experienced a major intestinal blockage that landed me in the hospital. I was scared to death at the possibility of removing more of my intestine. The blockage resolved itself after three days, and I went home determined that I would do everything in my power to find my way back to feeling healthy again.

The scans and bloodwork from the hospital showed other things as well though. I had a spot on my liver that they wanted to explore further, so I had two MRI's and an ultrasound with contrast dye. Nothing came from these as they determined that it was only scar tissue, either from years of inflamed colon or from one of my surgeries. My blood-work showed elevated levels of copper in my blood and a strange anomaly in one type of enzyme.

Thankfully, the copper levels went down on their own and the enzyme anomaly disappeared. Although extra liver testing showed nothing significant, I had an interesting conversation with the radiologist who performed my ultrasound.

"You're not cured," she declared after I vented my frustration with continuing to have so much pain after supposedly being cured from ulcerative colitis. "I wish the medical community would stop equating surgery with a cure. As an autoimmune disease, your cells are affected throughout your body. They don't stop at the large intestine. Inflammation can occur in other areas and you should start looking at what's causing the inflammation to begin with."

I felt validated. Strangely, I felt hopeful again. I didn't feel crazy for believing so strongly that the term "cured" was being used too flippantly.

Shortly after that enlightening visit, a follow-up with my GI doctor confirmed that my abdominal pain was related to scar tissue and also musculoskeletal in nature, meaning that it could be how my insides healed post-surgery. Following a pregnant pause he continued, "We can look at long-term pain management and prescriptions for painkillers if you need them."

Inside I was screaming, "Nooooo...!!" I couldn't imagine a lifetime of painkiller use ahead of me. I was 35 years old with three little kids at home. I was worried numbing that pain would numb other parts of my life as well.

I had a flashback to a nurse I had once chatted with in that same office, during the days of the clinical drug trial. She was a firm believer in the mix of western and eastern medicines. She had asked me if I had explored much yoga, meditation, or other forms of complementary medicine. At that time I had dabbled. I had tried a number of things, but didn't feel like I was successful at any approach to healing.

With that seed planted again, seven years after the initial conversation, a question from our innocent ten year old forced me to start taking this eastern medicine approach more seriously.

She came to me with a Guinness Book of World Records in hand, asking if I thought she would live longer than the oldest living person (who was currently 115 years old). "Maybe sweetie," I told her with a smile.

"How about you Mom? Imagine if we lived even longer than that - maybe I'll be 115 and you'll be 140."

"Oh my god!" I exclaimed, "There is absolutely no way. I don't even want to live past 70!"

A look of horror crossed her face and she asked me why. I struggled with trying to explain how difficult it was waking up every single morning in pain. Her poor ten year old heart had been hurt by my insistence on dying younger than normal. So, I recoiled my initial response and told her that the love in our family is much stronger than that pain and that I would want to live as long as possible to see her children, grandchildren, and great-grandchildren beyond that.

The truth of that – knowing how badly I really did want a life full of growing our family and making dreams become a reality - made me realize that I had to start taking my healing journey more seriously. The jungle analogy I gave earlier was very real. I felt completely lost among the pain and fatigue I was constantly experiencing, but I also felt certain that I could find better tools to help me find my way towards a place of healing.

My husband and kids deserved that. And although they were my motivation in the beginning of the journey, along the way I began to understand that I deserved it too.

Becoming a Map Maker

"For a star to be born, there is one thing that must happen:
a gaseous nebula must collapse. So collapse. Crumble.
This is not your destruction. This is your birth."
~ Zoe Skylar ~

When I started taking my quest to find health and healing seriously, I expected for things to click right away. I envisioned having one of those lightbulb moments, where I suddenly discovered the magic formula and then everything else would fall into place.

Not exactly how it turned out. I began trying different things and noticed improvements here and there, but more than anything it felt like I was constantly searching for the right path. My healing had started, but I was still lost in the jungle trying to find my way.

One thing I knew for certain was to explore the holistic connection between my Body, Mind, and Soul. So I added things into my life that I knew would benefit my overall well-being. I practiced more yoga, I saw a naturopath who helped me find better vitamins and supplements, I meditated more often, and I booked regular massages. It was definitely a start, but there was no real method to my madness. I was randomly exploring different things, wanting to try everything I could to find my way out of the jungle.

Then, tragedy struck. In September 2016, my oldest sister was diagnosed with terminal cancer. In the beginning we were told that she might have six months, and we held on to that number as a ray of hope, determined to make every day matter, every second count. Fate only gave us two of those months, and we lost our dear Vicki in November 2016, exactly five years after losing our dad to the same awful disease.

You don't really understand the term "heart-broken" until you actually experience it. Losing someone you love with all of your heart, with every part of your soul, shatters the world as you know it. It creates this hole inside of your heart, and during the most difficult days of grief, it feels like that hole is consuming you.

I found it difficult to move forward with my healing journey because on one hand it felt selfish and insignificant when I thought of everything my sister had endured. On the other hand, my motivation and ambition to find healing felt like it was lit on fire. My sister's sudden diagnosis and the ferocity of her cancer awoke the realization that life is short. We are never promised tomorrow. If I wanted change, I needed to make it happen today.

During that same fall, I attended a yoga retreat that I had booked months earlier. Eighteen of us spent two days at the Panther River Lodge, in the middle of nowhere, surrounded by mountains and a beautiful river. We were led by three amazing women through yoga, meditation, reiki, healing hands massage, sharing circles, a drumming ceremony, and quiet reflection.

Signing up for this retreat felt like one of the first times I had ever followed my heart. Something was calling me to this spot by the river, but truthfully all I was envisioning was a quiet weekend away with zero cell phone reception and some relaxing yoga. Instead I was given my first real sign that I was on the right path, and the awareness that greater healing was still ahead of me.

Through some raw and vulnerable sharing with complete strangers, enhanced by the healing powers of nature, I saw what was missing in my equation. I had been working towards healing my Body, Mind, and Soul; yet it was my Heart that needed to be tended to as well. Sitting by the edge of the river on my last day of the retreat, I felt the beginnings of true connections forming between my Body, Mind, Heart, and Soul.

The next part of my journey didn't proceed as smoothly or as directly as I would have liked. Knowing that my heart needed help while dealing with the loss of my sister, I reached out to a therapist who specialized in grief counselling. She taught me coping strategies, ways to honour my losses, and helped me give myself grace and understanding that grieving is a lifelong process. That was the easy part. Grief counselling morphed into everything-else counselling rather quickly, and for the first time ever I was learning how to take care of my emotional health.

This wasn't an easy road to travel down. I was working through emotions built up from the past 10 years, plus I was learning how to accept and work through new emotions that were bombarding me every day. My emotional health was volatile for a few weeks – I would erupt with anger or dissolve with sadness at a moment's notice. I felt like I had lost control. Healing my Heart was harder than I imagined.

This was in January 2017, and at this same time I was continuing to work on my health in other areas. My proper nutrition was giving me so much more energy and I was regularly working out. I was meditating every morning, I was decluttering my mind and my environment, and I was experiencing more focus and clarity than ever before. Then, as my emotions were all over the map, something strange started happening.

I began experiencing intestinal blockages. Four in the span of nine weeks. This is a problem that can be common among people with ostomies, especially if we're not being careful about what we're eating or how well we're chewing our food. However, I was being vigilant about both of those things.

A blockage usually starts out as partial where you experience cramping, bloating and gas. Sometimes I can help it move along through stretching, a hot bath, a heating pad, walking around, or believe it or not, drinking a can of Coke. When it gets worse, the pain becomes intense, nausea takes over, and I become dehydrated quickly as I can't consume anything without vomiting. At this point I need to get to a hospital right away to receive IV hydration and anti-nausea medication, which is often enough to get the blockage moving. I am usually sent home that same day with instructions for a temporary liquid diet.

My blockages worked themselves out with the help of these ER visits, but my doctors were confused about what could be causing them if it wasn't diet. The general consensus was that it would likely be a buildup of scar tissue in my small intestine from so much inflammation over the years. It was like having a kink in a garden hose.

I was discouraged because I felt like I was on the right path by intentionally working on my physical, mental, emotional, and spiritual health. Yet, these major potholes on my journey felt like they were really setting me back.

This was when I first realized how interconnected everything was. When one area of my health was out of balance, it quickly created a snowball effect and plowed into the other areas causing negative side effects and challenges along the way.

My Body was struggling with constant intestinal blockages. I was having a lot of trouble sleeping, and when I did sleep it didn't feel restful. My nutrition was impacted as the liquid and mush diet I had to consume wasn't giving me the energy I needed. I gave up on exercising, or even doing yoga because it was all so difficult.

With my physical health out of whack, my Mind struggled next. I couldn't stay focused or on task as I tried juggling a hundred different thoughts and ideas. I felt overwhelmed, unsettled, and indecisive. So, my mental health was off-kilter as the snowball plowed into my Mind.

My Heart was a giant mess, as I worked through the emotional breakdown I was experiencing. In fact, I wonder if the snowball didn't start here. My emotional upheaval might have been the root problem that began the snowball effect into other areas. Feelings of confusion, doubt, worry, and frustration took over the space in my Heart.

Now, with my Body, Mind, and Heart all in disarray, they took my Soul right along with them for the ride. Everything was in such a state of imbalance that I lost my connection to myself and the bigger picture. My Soul was becoming clouded with the unanswerable question *"why me?"* and I was losing faith in my Body's ability to become healthy again.

Fortunately, I realized that this snowball effect was hurting every part of my well-being, and I was determined to take control of the situation again. I decided to start adding small changes back into my life, intentionally working on my Body, Mind, Heart, and Soul. I revisited my nutritionist, and started seeing a pelvic physiotherapist. I had a few reiki sessions and participated in my first breath workshop. I forced myself to go to bed earlier and reconnected with meditation and simple, restorative yoga routines.

I knew that too much would be overwhelming so I kept it simple, doing small things consistently to help keep my focus on taking care of my health and well-being. My strength came back in my Body, and with it my Heart and my Soul suddenly felt stronger than they ever had before. My Mind followed suit as well, as some of the tools I was using were having a ripple effect through every part of me.

The lightbulb never went off in that sudden "aha" moment of discovery, yet there was no doubt that I was on to something that was working wonders in my life. Mike noticed some of the changes right away, as did the kids. While we were cooking together one afternoon, my oldest daughter commented "Mom, you look really happy..." My heart burst with appreciation for her noticing, but I also felt the sting of realizing how much hurt and exhaustion my family had witnessed throughout my years of pain and fatigue.

Friends and family were next to notice and then a few doctor's visits showed me that these results were taking hold in other ways as well. My inflammatory markers were way down and those kinks in my intestine were not showing up in exams. Suddenly, I realized how several weeks had passed without feeling that incessant, painful knot in my side.

Pain-free? I couldn't remember the last time that I was pain-free. Whatever I was doing was working. What was I doing? It seemed to be a hodgepodge collection of habits that I had collected over the course of time. I sat down with a giant sketchpad of my kids and started drawing a spider web of what I was doing and what was working.

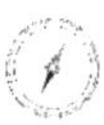

My Healing Compass was born. I realized that I had been dividing my healthy activities between my Body, Mind, Heart, and Soul. I also realized that my method of tracking and monitoring those habits was working very well for me. As I drew and sketched a more formal version of what this Healing Compass looked like to me, I became more and more excited about using it long-term.

I felt like I had finally found my way out of the jungle. Over time I had collected the best tools possible for achieving my balanced state of health and wellness. Better than that, I had discovered something more significant – **how** to use those tools to find healing in every area of my life. I had officially become a mapmaker.

I created a template that I use to assess my overall health in each of the four areas at the beginning of every month. And I developed a simple habit tracker to be more consistent about using my tools as often as possible.

Three months later, it became clear to me that this really was working in my life. My Body felt strong with increased energy, my Mind was clear and focused, my Heart was more connected than ever before, and my Soul suddenly felt a sense of drive and purpose.

This little fire in my Soul was first lit back at that yoga retreat the previous fall. Now it was ready to spread into action, making my dreams and vision come true. I always had a dream of writing a book, and for a long time I felt like my purpose in life was to help others. What would happen if I combined the two?

Here we are, with *The Healing Compass.* I want to share what I've learned, and how I use that knowledge to live my life to the fullest. I've never felt healthier or happier than I do right now, and I wish that everyone could find that same health and happiness in their lives. Incorporating your Healing Compass into your life will help you find your own unique path to optimal health and happiness in your Body, Mind, Heart, and Soul.

The Compass

Building your Healing Compass will give you the forward momentum you need to start taking better care of your Body, Mind, Heart, and Soul. As you learn to start taking care of your whole self, you will move from a place of surviving to thriving, from feeling stuck to moving intentionally towards living life to the fullest.

The best part is that this whole process and practice is neither complicated nor time consuming. You will weave two themes throughout the creation of your personal Compass:

1. **Keep It Simple:** Really simple. When you add a new habit or tweak an existing one, it doesn't have to be complicated or confusing. Repeat the mantra "Keep it Simple" anytime you start to feel overwhelmed.

2. **Small Changes can lead to Huge Results:** It's beautiful that you don't need to tackle a huge overhaul in your life to

start seeing forward momentum. Tiny changes can make a big impact.

How can small changes make such a huge difference? With the addition of two important ingredients:

1. **Consistency:** It's important to check-in with your Compass every morning and night. To build healthy habits into your life, you need to plan and monitor the tiny changes you are making.
2. **Intention:** You won't change any part of your life if you don't want to put in the effort. Remember, I'm not talking about monumental changes, but instead focusing on simple habits to help you heal. Intention comes with commitment and following through with these daily check-ins.

I promise that you will fail if you don't take these ingredients seriously, and I can also promise that you will see major results if you fully embrace them.

The Compass has four quadrants to it:

Body = Physical Health

Mind = Intellectual Health

Heart = Emotional Health

Soul = Spiritual Health

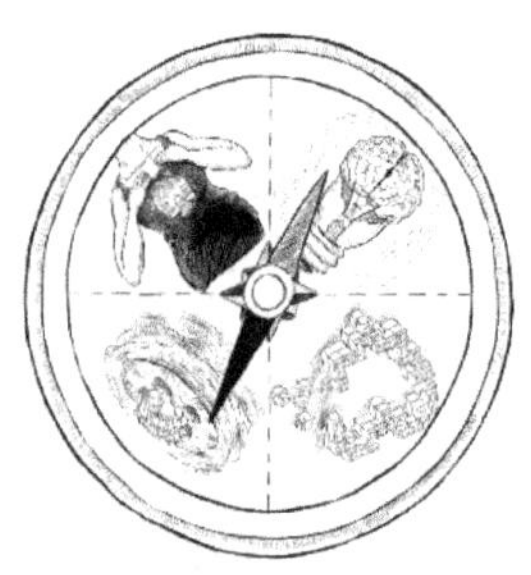

Your main goal is to find *your* unique path towards feeling healthier and happier. Once you feel the deep-rooted connection between your Body, Mind, Heart, and Soul, your life will feel more whole and fulfilled than ever before. To find that path, and build your own map you will learn how to use the Compass and its sidekick the Tracker.

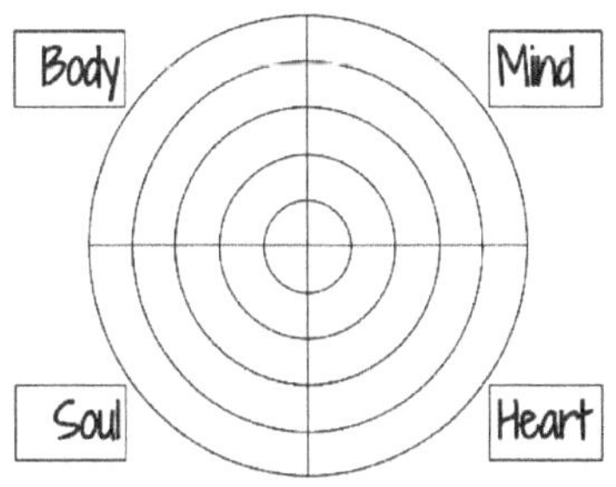

The Compass: This is where you assess yourself at the beginning of each month to see how you're doing and determine where you need to focus more time.

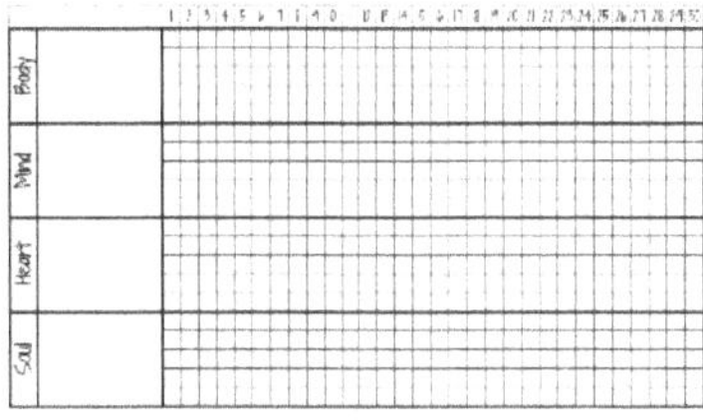

The Tracker: This is where you check-in daily to remind yourself of the healthy habits you're building into your life.

And these are the basic steps you follow:

- **Assess:** Reflect at the beginning of the month on how you're feeling in your Body, Mind, Heart, and Soul.
- **Monitor:** Check-in every morning and every night to cross off what you've accomplished.
- **Repeat:** If something isn't working you can always change it and adapt.

This book is broken up into four sections. Each one discusses a corner of the Compass and walks through five key habits that you can focus on to help bring balance and better health to your life.

Within each chapter and habit we talk about:

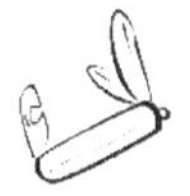

Your Tools:

→ The practical things you can do in your everyday life to help make this habit take hold.

And...

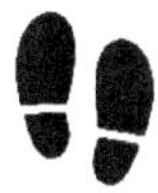

Your Next Steps:

→ One or two simple things you can do, starting today to make these changes start happening.

It took an army of mentors and outside inspiration to get me to this place in my life and I'm forever grateful for all of the help I've had along the way. I share these mentors with you in hopes that they'll inspire some of you as well. You'll see this throughout the book:

Inspired By...

Name of Brilliant Person... and how they helped me find my path to health and happiness.

I also want to provide the support and encouragement to get more out of a particular area for anyone needing that extra push in their lives. In the introduction of each section (Body, Mind, Heart, and Soul) you will find a segment called **Bring Out the Backhoe.** It looks like this:

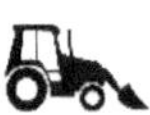

Bring Out the Backhoe...

How to dig deeper into a particular subject when you need and want more...

The backhoe is in reference to my amazing dad, who I miss with every fiber of my being. He was a backhoe operator and whenever I feel myself "digging deeper" into any particular area of my life, a smile comes to my face as I visualize my dad behind the wheel of his backhoe with a big grin.

Here is a quick glimpse at the printable which includes the

Compass and Tracker. You can find your free copy (in colour) at:
www.myhealingcompass.com/compass

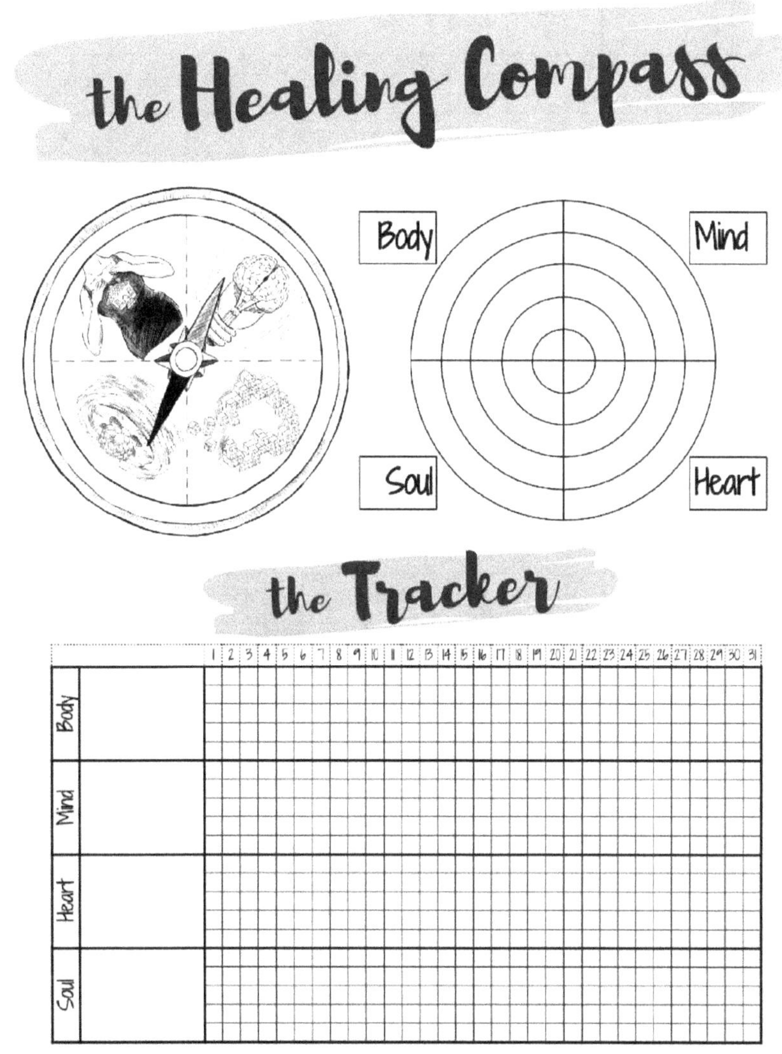

You will learn exactly how to work with your Compass and Tracker when you get to the chapter *Your Compass* at the end of this book. For now, here are a few examples of what the tracker looks like filled out.

In the beginning, your Tracker might look like this at the end of the month:

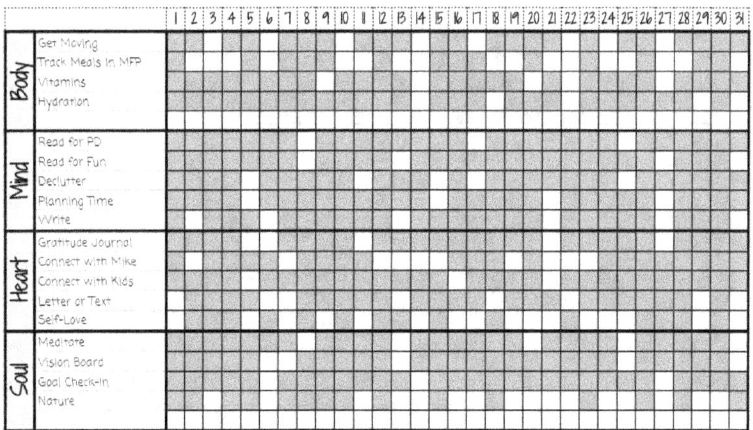

Notice that we only start with one or two things in each area of the Compass. Over time we might choose to add more and it may look more like this:

Every month will be different because life is constantly changing. As seasons change and life events happen, the areas of our health that we need to focus on will shift as well. Some months we need to take a step back and focus on less things, but more intently. Other months our energy and motivation allow us to work on more areas of our health with drive and ambition.

We will discuss more specifics about setting up your own

Healing Compass after we get through the four sections. Remember the key to success is to **Keep it Simple.** As you read through the chapters, you may feel tempted to start implementing a bunch of changes right away. We know that won't work. The importance is a balance between our Body, Mind, Heart, and Soul; and to start small and simple.

"If the ladder is not leaning against the right wall, every step we take just gets us to the wrong place faster."
~ Stephen Covey ~

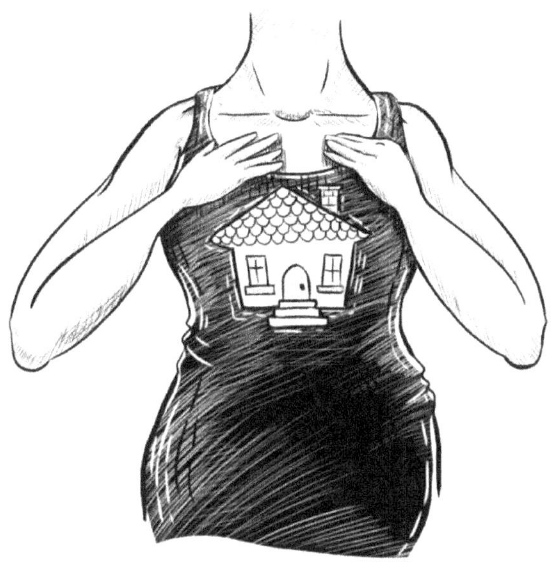

Your Body

(Section One)

"A wise man ought to realize that health is
his most valuable possession."
~ *Hippocrates* ~

It's important to start with healing your Body because your physical health gives you the foundation for everything else in life. It becomes impossible to work on your Mind, Heart, and Soul when this area is out of balance.

Whether you're struggling with illness or feeling healthy, taking care of the one and only body you have should be your main focus every single day. Would you spend hours polishing the leather inside your vehicle and searching for the best scent of air freshener, if the engine itself was falling apart and was ready to leave you stranded on the side of the road?

"Take care of your body. It's the only place you have to live."
~ Jim Rohn ~

The biggest challenge is that the world around us makes it harder to stay focused on our physical health than ever before. Think about it - all day, every day, you have a zillion options enabling you to choose crappy food and sit on the couch all day long.

Have you ever been caught in a social media rabbit hole? Or maybe found yourself plunked on that couch watching mindless TV for hours on end. Not to mention the equally insane amount of poor food choices that are at your disposal any time of day or night. 24-hour drive-thrus? Can you believe how busy those can be at 2:00 a.m.? Why do we need the luxury of buying processed junk at that time in the morning?

In theory it all sounds so easy...

- Be active & eat nutritious foods
- Get the proper amount of sleep
- Take care of your body and it will take care of you

Yet there are millions of us struggling with this each and every day. When our other areas of the compass are out of balance, we tend to view our physical health as being too complicated or complex to figure out.

You may say things like: "I'll find time for it later... when I'm feeling better." Or, "I'll start eating better on Monday, I promise."

How many Mondays go by without that happening? I had to change my mindset and believe these two truths about my Body in order to become unstuck:

- I have to take care of myself *now.*
- No one else will do it for me.

"The trouble is, you think you have time..."
~ *Jack Kornfield* ~

As you start learning how to make your physical health a priority, the wheels are set in motion so that you can start tackling the other areas next. When your Body has more energy, your Mind begins to have more focus and clarity, your Heart begins to grow with pride and confidence, and your Soul becomes alive with peace and purpose.

What are you going to work on in this section?

Let's Get Moving - Move your body. Every day. In a way that works for you.
Eat Like Great Grandma - Start viewing food as fuel for your day. Believe that it can make or break how well your body functions, and cut out the junk. For real.
Catch Those Zzzz's - Make sleep a priority and not an afterthought. Learn the tools you need to give your body the rest that it desperately needs to heal.
Tune into Your Body - Learn what you can about what those various aches and pains mean. Listen to the cues your body is sending you.
Build Your Health Posse - Take charge of learning more about what can help you. Find the perfect recipe for Eastern and Western Medicine.

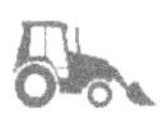 Bring Out the Backhoe...

Whole 30 – cofounded by Melissa Hartwig:
In the simplest of definitions, this is a 30 day clean-eating plan that gives your body a break from foods that can have a negative impact on your health. In the words of Melissa, this program is a way of pushing the reset button on our bodies. The premise is simple. You remove grains, dairy, legumes, sugar, alcohol, and all processed junk from your meals for a full 30 days. No cheat meals are allowed because your body needs to have those items eliminated completely for a month in order to add them back in and see which, if any foods, may be causing you trouble. These foods, especially in excess, have been linked to inflammation, gut issues, hormonal problems, and more. There's no calorie counting and no weighing yourself. You're encouraged to focus on what they call "non-scale victories" – things like better sleep, less pain, more energy, clear skin, etc. When 30 days have passed, you systematically reintroduce those foods individually to see if you experience any side effects (bloating, cramping, or general yuckiness). Then hopefully, you continue on with your life having formed a better relationship with food. You will know which foods might be causing you problems, and then you can decide if it's worth it *to you* to bring them back into your life. Your body doesn't like sugar? You can still say "yes" to that chocolate cupcake that's calling your name on your birthday, just be aware of the negative effects it has if you continue eating it on a regular basis. You can make healthy, conscious decisions about what you put into your body, asking yourself "do I *really* want this? Or is it a temporary craving?" The Whole 30 program can change your life by helping you better understand which foods are harming you and which foods are healing you.

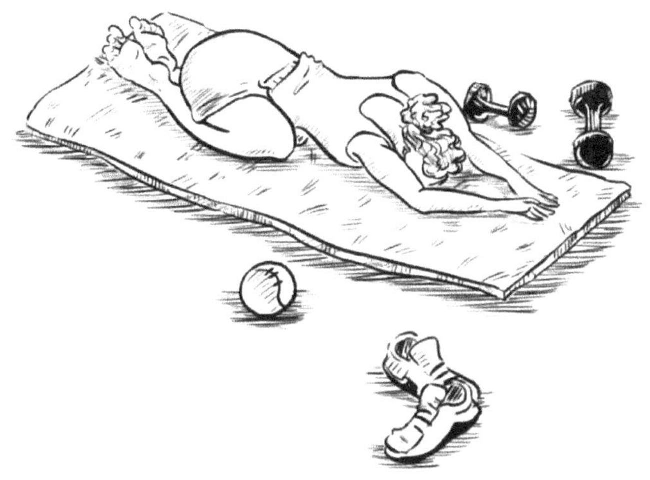

Let's Get Moving

"Exercise is a celebration of what your body
can do. Not a punishment for what you ate."
~ Unknown ~

Is there anyone else out there that's become incredibly gifted at the art of coming up with excuses about why you can't exercise today? Or is it just me?

"My knees hurt. My head hurts. My *insert body part* hurts. I'll start tomorrow. I'll start Monday. I have to get this laundry done first. I have to reply to that email first. I'm in a rough stretch. It's been a rough day. It's a full moon - should you exercise on a full moon?"

Also, it turns out that one of my biggest downfalls in life is that I'm a planner much more than I am a doer. This is how, over the course of one month, I accumulated 294 images and links on my "Get Moving" Pinterest board, and very few steps on my fitness tracker. I seriously thought that finding a huge selection of fitness ideas, programs, challenges, and motivational quotes was going to get me moving.

Is it shocking news to tell you that it didn't work? But I did have a lightbulb moment that finally got my butt in gear.

I saw this quote:

"Comparison is the thief of joy"
~ *Theodore Roosevelt* ~

The quote was on social media and after I scrolled past it, I immediately saw a picture of one of my amazing cousins completing a marathon. I have a whole slew of crazy cousins who do things like "run for fun" and test themselves with 100 mile races.

"I wish I could do that..." - the thought drifted through my mind. Then I remembered the comparison quote and CLICK, the lightbulb turned on. I realized that I had been comparing my physical fitness abilities to every single person around me, both in real life and online. It's not that I was aspiring to become a runner, but in my head I had set a standard for physical activity and it more or less had to be all or nothing.

The bar I had set for myself was a 30 minute walk, at least 5 days a week. And I was failing miserably. That sounds so simple now - a 30 minute walk every day. Have you been there though? Stuck in the flawed logic of "if I can't do it all the way, then I won't do it at all..." mixed with the toxic second thought of "I'll do it later, there's always tomorrow."

"There's always tomorrow" is a double edged sword. It has some useful applications, but more often than not it is our justification for procrastinating. In short, I needed a mindset shift. I had to change my inflexible expectations to something realistic and easy to manage.

To help set realistic goals, let's change the definition of being active to this: Not sitting still. You can add physical activity to your life every single day by choosing to simply get off your butt more often than not.

It also helps to understand that what works for some people might not work for you. You will need to keep trying and searching and trying some more until you find the right activities that click for you.

For myself, I needed to start small. I took baby steps, and as I began sprinkling more and more little bouts of activity into my life, the more I wanted. My motivation and confidence shot up as I wanted to push myself a little bit more each day. There are no 100 mile marathons in my future, but I feel great about tackling those beginner hikes in the mountains, and I feel fantastic about my physical self continuing to become stronger and healthier.

I honestly started with some basics. I would walk to get the mail - it was only a block away, and then I started taking the long way home. I parked farther away in parking lots to get some extra steps in. I played with my kids more, whether it was catch in the backyard or having an impromptu dance party in the living room. Small steps started leading to big changes.

"Little by little, one travels far."
~ J.R.R. Tolkien ~

What holds us back from taking those small steps, little by little, is generally an unhealthy mix of fear, comparison, and self-doubt. If you find yourself in the "not enough" mindset, you will never move forward.

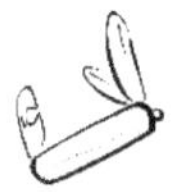

Your Tools:

→ **Stop Comparing:** Easier said than done, right? Nine times out of ten we don't even realize that we're doing it, but Constant Comparison Complex seems to prevent most of us from taking those first steps forward.

→ **Use the Internet for Good:** There are many reasons to dislike that world-wide web, but one wonderful thing about it is that you can very easily find a workout program that works for you. Try *Fitness Blender* for a whole schwack of amazing, free workout videos. Yoga lovers can try out *Yoga with Adrienne.* Her YouTube channel is full of routines of every shape and size and her laid-back nature makes it feel like a friend is teaching you the ins and outs of yoga.

→ **Combine Physical Activity with Something You Enjoy:** I learned this habit-forming strategy from Gretchen Rubin's book *Better Than Before,* and this is how I use it:
   o I watch a favourite show on Netflix while I'm on the treadmill and commit to only watching it while working out so that I have more motivation to get moving.[1]
   o I spend an hour pulling weeds in the garden. Combining movement with Vitamin D from the sun and feeling spiritually grounded by connecting with nature? Totally win-win.

→ **Monitor Progress in a Fun Way:** I love my fitness tracker and find that it definitely helps motivate me, but before it, pen and paper also worked well. I would set a goal, usually a distance that I wanted to travel, and then draw that distance out with boxes so that I could fill in the distance that I

---

[1] Thank you Gilmore Girls for helping me lose 15 lbs this year!

covered. For example, I once wanted to walk the distance from Calgary to Vancouver (982 km) over the span of 5 months. I'd track my steps daily through a phone app and try to see how far I could get!

→ **Remember to Keep it Simple:** You will achieve much greater success if you don't over-plan, overthink, or set too high of expectations. On a day when you don't feel like doing that workout or yoga session, just dance! Throw on a happy song and bebop[2] around the living room for 5 minutes.

"Remember, a 30 minute workout is just 2% of your day."
~ Unknown ~

I can't stress it enough - find something that works for you, something that gets you excited about being active. I know it's out there somewhere.

 **Inspired By...**

Peace in a Pod Yoga: For the longest time, I did yoga on and off. I found that I enjoyed it, but I never *loved* it. Friends would rave about this yoga studio or that yoga studio and I would always leave feeling disappointed because I felt so inferior to all of the well-toned, agile yogis out there. Nothing ever completely clicked for me. Until one day, I found my yoga studio - a place where I felt no inferiority or comparison, and when I left my first yoga session there, it felt like I was walking on air. Now isn't it ironic that when I lived in a city of over one million people I tried time and time again, but couldn't find a place that clicked with me? Yet, when we moved to a rural area I found my yoga studio in a town of one thousand people. Peace in a Pod Yoga is a place where you'll find yogis of every age and ability and the overall

---

2 Only if you have an old soul. I hear young souls don't bee-bop. Their loss...

---

atmosphere is so homey and welcoming.

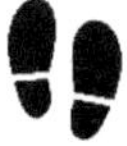 # *Your Next Steps:*

→ Write a list of simple, active ideas that you can try. Things that you can easily add into your day, and make an effort to do one of those things each and every day.

→ Pick something new to try, whether it's a class at a gym or studio, or something you find online. Put it on the calendar, at least two times this week. Don't cancel that appointment with yourself for anything.

"No matter how slow you go, you're still lapping
everybody on the couch."
~ Unknown ~

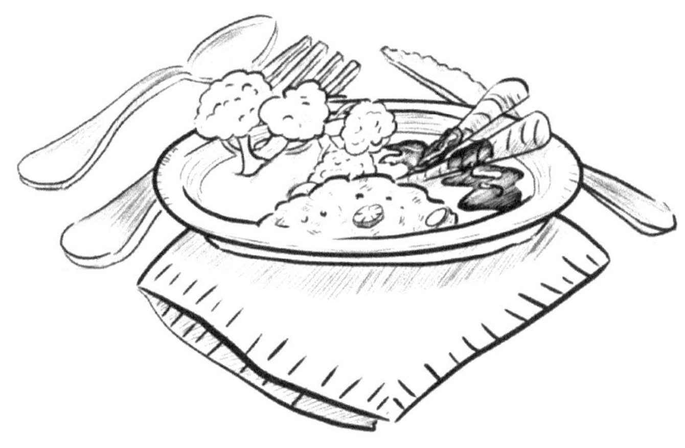

Eat Like Great-Grandma

"What you find at the end of your fork is more powerful than anything you'll find at the bottom of a pill bottle."
~ Mary Buchan ~

I love to cook, I adore cooking shows, and I have a slight addiction to buying cookbooks. The kitchen has become my happy place - where I go to ease stress and do something that fuels my soul.

I know it's not that way for everyone. Whether or not you like spending time in the kitchen, the nitty-gritty of using nutrition to heal ourselves is one of the simplest changes we can make.

My love for cooking is very real, but so is my love/hate relationship with food. Suffering from a digestive disorder, and living with a permanent ostomy, I've really had to dig deep into figuring out what foods cause me trouble and what foods help heal inflammation.

The reality is that many of us need to educate ourselves more on which foods are helping us and which are harming us. The food industry has tricked us for years, with making sure that the most addictive food products are marketed in a way to make them appear healthy.

You'll see "all natural", "vitamin fortified", and even "made with whole grains" on food packages all around you. Most of those products are packed full of preservatives and high amounts of sugar. A lot of people believe that they're making the right choice reaching for that container of zero-fat yogurt, not knowing that it's jam packed with sugar and chemically engineered ingredients.

"If it comes from a plant, eat it.
If it was made in a plant, don't."
~ Michael Pollan ~

Before our grocery stores became over-run with all of the boxes, cans, and bags that come from a factory instead of a farm, people ate real food. We need to get back to that. Think about your Great-Grandma and the food that she would have ate - vegetables grown in her garden, meat locally produced and butchered, and bread baked from scratch.

That might sound complicated, but it's not. Eating real food doesn't mean you have to start baking your own bread and growing all of your own vegetables. You can get real foods made with real ingredients from your local grocery store or Farmer's Market. Eating like Great-Grandma means moving away from factory produced foods and moving towards non-manufactured food.

Depending on where you're at in your food journey, the idea of eating real food can be overwhelming to those who live off of the convenience of processed and fast foods. Just think of taking baby steps. Keep it simple and start small.

I started by finding some recipes with real food ingredients that I wanted to try. I cooked them, my family loved them, and I kept going from there. We cleaned out our pantry and got rid of the cans and boxes of things that were loaded with ingredients whose names we couldn't pronounce.[3] We made a big effort to start eating more fruits and veggies. We started becoming regulars at the local Farmer's Market and began purchasing our meat from local farms whose animal raising and grazing practices we were familiar with.

"A healthy outside starts from the inside."
~ *Robert Urich* ~

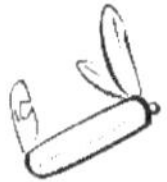 *Your Tools:*

→ **Read Labels:** This can feel like a real chore sometimes. I just want to get into the grocery store and back out again. So, the first thing I do is try to eat food that doesn't have labels! Then, for the small amount of things we use that are canned or boxed (pasta, coconut milk, some spices), I've found a brand that works and always keep it stock piled.

---

[3] Bye-bye neon green chicken noodle soup and orange mac & cheese...

→ **Meal Planning & Prepping:** This is a big one. It'll be easier to stick to eating real foods and wholesome meals if your meals are planned ahead of time. You won't be tempted to grab something quick en route because you already have dinner planned and ready to whip up when you get home. Even better is when you can prepare meals for the freezer in order to have lots of healthy, ready to cook meals at your fingertips. It's perfect for those times when it would just be so much easier to phone for take-out.

→ **Progress, not Perfection:** Do we still eat fast food occasionally? I'm not going to lie, we do...but it's rare. Not to mention, after my taste-buds have changed fast food just doesn't taste good anymore. Do we splurge on a bag of chips or donuts once in a while? Absolutely. Are they made with 100% real food ingredients? Not likely. Over 90% of our meals are real food based, and that's a benchmark that I'm happy to meet.

"When you start eating food without labels,
you no longer need to count calories."
~ *Amanda Kraft* ~

My favourite part about striving to eat like Great Grandma is that it isn't a fad diet, or the latest trend for losing weight. Instead it's a forever plan, a new lifestyle that makes you feel so much better, inside and out. As you begin putting more real food into your body and continue removing factory-made chemical concoctions from your diet, you will notice big changes.

 **Inspired By…**

Rory Hornstein, RD (Calgary, AB): I feel like I have found the best dietician/ nutritionist on the planet. She's the third one I have met with, so if this is a step that is important to you (primarily if you have digestive issues of any kind), know that you can keep trying until you find someone that you click with. One of the best things about her is that she also has IBD, so when we're talking about foods that cause me trouble and hurt to digest, she gets it - 100%. Plus she has this amazing personality and hilarious sense of humour, so I leave our visits with a huge smile on my face. And she cares - deeply, truly cares about the wellbeing of her clients. Just when I'm starting to feel like I'm in a bit of a funk, I receive an email in my inbox from Rory, "just checking in".

100 Days of Real Food: Lisa Leake is a leading expert on the area of real food, and her simple, back to the basics approach is refreshing. I have both of her cookbooks on my shelf (she's working on a third!), and we've made and enjoyed pretty much every single recipe from those pages. Her website is full of useful information and she does an amazing job of showing us how making a shift to whole-food cooking doesn't have to break the bank.

Against All Grain: Danielle Walker is a food blogger, cookbook author, and genuine amazing human being. I have identified with her for a long time because she also has Ulcerative Colitis and has helped heal herself through choosing the right foods, and eliminating the wrong foods. I am also obsessed with her cookbooks. I'm currently cooking my way through each one and I am so excited that she's coming out with a fourth this year!

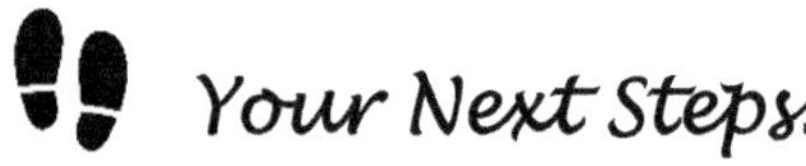 # *Your Next Steps:*

→ Make a list of real foods and meals with real ingredients that you love. Think back to the basics - spaghetti and meatballs, shepherd's pie, roast chicken, and veggies.

→ Start adding those meals into your regular meal routine.

→ Pay attention to what you're buying at the grocery store - is it real food? Or is it processed with a list of ingredients you can't pronounce?

→ Make progress each day, without stressing about perfection. Be intentional about the food you're putting into your body.

"The food you eat can be either the safest and most powerful form of medicine, or the slowest form of poison."
~ Ann Wigmore ~

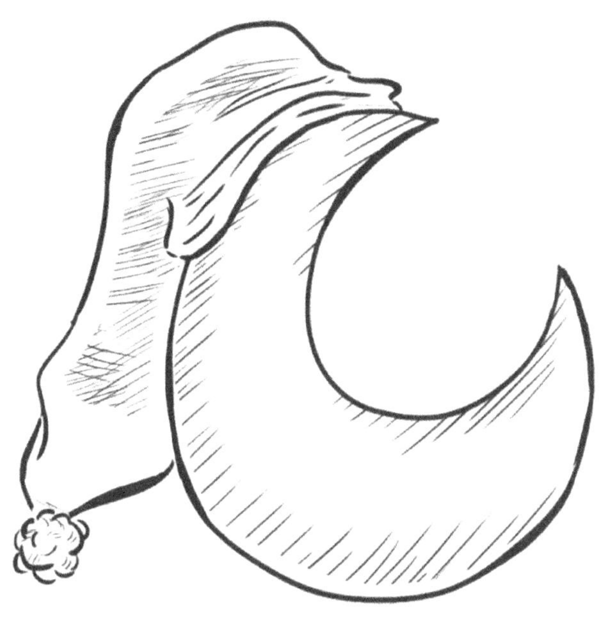

Catch Those Zzzz's

"My eyelids are heavy.
But my thoughts are heavier."
~ Unknown ~

I used to dread sleep. Like more than doing laundry. That's serious dread. We probably had this mutual dislike of each other because I treated it so poorly, and sleep didn't give me much in return. I spent years tossing and turning.

Sleep didn't come very easily because to-do lists were always swirling around in my brain and the very act of laying down in bed acted as a conduit for 27 more things to jump on to that list. For years my body was in so much pain that sleep didn't stick around for long either. I would wake up at least every hour on the hour, uncomfortable and irritated that I had to try and fall back asleep again.

I hated the next part just as much - getting out of bed. I loved to hit the snooze button half a dozen times, or moan and groan at the kids that were trying to drag me out of bed at the crack of dawn, begging them to just go and turn on a cartoon.

The first problem in this whole scenario was that I was treating sleep as the enemy. I put it off as long as humanly possible, justifying my staying up late because I needed "me time". That was just a fancy excuse because I didn't usually use the time for filling up my self-care cup. I would often be working, catching up on emails, mindlessly browsing the internet, or even hustling to finish housework.

Then I would crash into our bed, often wearing the same comfy pants and t-shirt that I had worn all day, and many times completely skipping the face washing and teeth brushing portion of the evening.

No wonder sleep didn't grace me with its presence. I was a brutal host of the party. I saw sleep as a necessary evil that was interrupting my desire to watch more, read more, and do more. Oh, how wrong I was.

"You're still a ROCKSTAR", I whisper to myself
as I take a multivitamin and go to bed at 9:45"
~ Unknown ~

I read a book called *The Sleep Revolution* by Ariana Huffington and it changed my views on sleep forever. I stopped making excuses about why I needed to stay up a little bit longer and I quit trying to cram more and more into my days, avoiding rest in the process.

Most of all, I started paying close attention to the idea of sleep hygiene, even though I didn't believe it was a real 'thing' at first. Sleep hygiene? How hokey does that sound? But as I started building these tools of sleep hygiene into my life, suddenly my rest actually felt rejuvenating. My mornings were filled with energy instead of me dreading them beginning. As I appreciated everything my body was doing for me during those important hours of rest, it seemed like my body was repaying me with more energy, less mood swings, and better health.

"A good laugh and a long sleep are
the two best cures for anything."
~ *Irish Proverb* ~

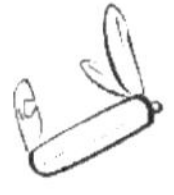 ## Your Tools:

→ **Set the Scene:** Sleep craves a dark room, without so much as a night light or even the red glow of an alarm clock. Think 'middle-of-the-woods" dark. Also, cool temperatures. You can be snuggled under as many blankets as you'd like, but the ambient temperature of the room should be around 18 degrees Celsius or 65 degrees Fahrenheit. And finally, sleep comes better with quiet. Which can be difficult because some noise in our bedroom is within our control and some isn't.[4] We can't control the cars driving by or the sirens in the distance, but we can drown them out with white noise. There are apps we can download on our phones or machines we can purchase for very little money.

---

[4] Ahem... snoring partners.

→ **Set a Bedtime:** Treat yourself like you would a 2 year old. I am fanatical about getting my kids to bed on time, and I realized that I deserved the same approach. Figure out your wake-up time and make your go-to-bed time by counting 7-8 hours backwards. Easy peasy. Even try setting a "go-to-bed" alarm the same way you would set a "wake-up" alarm. Set it a little bit ahead of when you want to fall asleep so that you can actually unwind before catching those zzzz's.

→ **Unwind:** Get the boring stuff out of the way first - washing your face and brushing your teeth. Do you ever find yourself procrastinating going to bed just because you don't feel like getting ready for bed? Bonus Tip: You're less likely to do that dreaded late night snacking after your teeth are sparkly clean and minty fresh! Next, do something that relaxes and calms you before you turn out the lights. Try one of these on for size:

- meditating	- journal writing	- reading
- stretching	- gentle yoga	- soothing music

→ **Pyjamas or your Birthday Suit:** That's right, your call because either work. Just stop climbing into bed wearing the same clothes you work-out in, or the same comfy clothes you wear around the house all day long.[5] In the book, *The Sleep Revolution* I learned that actual bed-clothes "send a signal to our brain that it is time to shut down." I never would have believed this to be true until I tried it out myself. As I found myself feeling sleepier and falling asleep quickly, this became a part of my ritual that I never skip out on.

"Without enough sleep, we all become tall two year olds."
~ JoJo Jensen ~

The more I studied sleep habits and dug into the research on

---

[5] I'm looking at you comfy yoga pants and old college t-shirt.

how poor sleep was negatively impacting my life, I quickly became obsessed with improving it. I realized the cost of poor sleep was substantial. It was affecting my:

Body - putting me at greater risk for stroke, heart disease, dementia, and some cancers, while also weakening my immune system.
Mind - my memory and basic ability to process thoughts and actions becomes impaired with lack of sleep.
Heart - anxiety and stress levels increase, along with the likelihood of feeling depressed.

As I read more information on sleep, one major theme became clear - the smartest and most successful people in our society also have strict and similar sleep rituals and schedules. Coincidence? I don't think so. Sleep is incredibly important in helping us live our lives to the fullest and achieving all of our dreams.

The best part is that proper sleep will lead to substantial growth in other areas of your life. You'll choose healthier foods, you'll have more energy for exercise, you'll discover more patience in your relationships, you'll be able to stay more focused on your daily tasks... the list goes on.

 **Inspired By...**

Arianna Huffington: Her book *The Sleep Revolution* had a huge impact on the views I have regarding sleep. She talks at great length about how our terrible relationship with sleep is causing profound consequences in so many areas of our lives. She offers many more tips than I provide here and digs in deep to some of the science and psychology around sleep, or our lack of it.

👣 *Your Next Steps:*

→ Pick one or two things from the list of tools to try at first. Just one or two.

→ Try them consistently for a week, and then add one or two more things and try those for a week.

→ **Keep it simple.** These are simple changes and easy tasks that will lead to amazing, healthy sleep habits.

"The amount of sleep required by the average person
is five minutes more."
~ *Unknown* ~

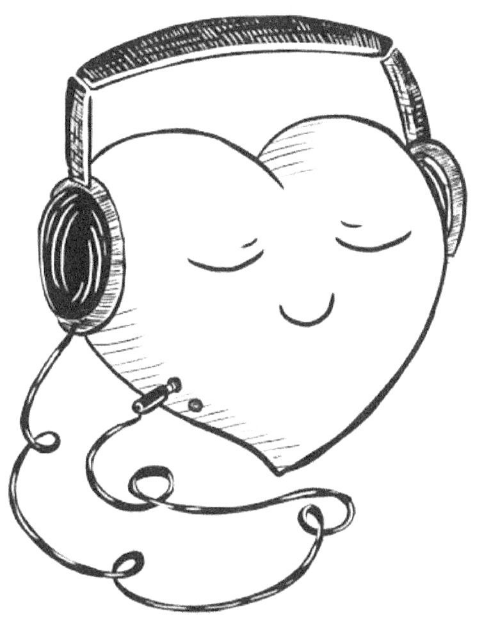

Tune Into Your Body

"If you listen to your body when it whispers,
you won't have to hear it scream."
~ Unknown ~

Out of all of the relationships that I've had to learn to navigate, my relationship with my body has been a very challenging one. For a long time, it was a rather abusive relationship instead of being patient, loving, and nurturing.

Let's see... I often treated sleep as a major inconvenience, inhaled whatever food I could grab the quickest, sat around in a computer chair for too many hours out of the day, and grabbed the closest bottle of Tylenol every time my head started to throb.

I was pushing my body to the brink of a breakdown. Perhaps the worst thing I did was chain myself to a limiting belief that plagued me for 13 years. When my body started breaking down as chronic illness took over, I kept repeating this defeating story to myself: "This isn't fair. I'm only 24. Why is my body doing this to me?"

That number changed every year as I repeated the mantra with each birthday that passed. Then I stopped at 37. I finally realized and believed that my body wasn't to blame. We were in this together, for better or worse.

"Sometimes when you're in a dark place, you think you've been buried, but actually you've been planted."
~ Unknown ~

As respect for my body grew, I learned more about my illness and the symptoms I was experiencing. I was able to move from constantly ignoring my body, to responding to the signals it was sending me.

Respect came from reflecting on everything my body was doing for me every single day. Your body is working all day, every day, without a single break. Even when you're sleeping your cells are regenerating, blood is pumping throughout your body, your liver is cleansing toxins, and nutrients are being absorbed to fuel you with more energy. If you don't stop to actually think about the incredible machine your body is, taking it for granted comes rather naturally.

I also realized that my body doesn't send warning signs or smoke signals to anyone else on the planet. Just me. I am officially in charge of making my health and healing a priority, and I can trust that my body is filled with infinite wisdom about what it needs.

My body gives me all sorts of signals now that I've learned to slow down and listen to what it has to say. When my patience is wearing thin and I'm easily irritated, chances are my body is requesting some healthy food and not just a quick snack to try and tide it over.[6] When I'm yawning over and over and over again, I don't need to push myself through one more hour of writing or catching up on housework. I need to rest.

"I listen to my body, it knows exactly what I need."
~ Kris Carr ~

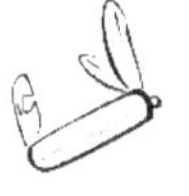 ## Your Tools:

→ **Become the Expert:** If you have a physical or mental illness, become knowledgeable on what exactly is going on inside of your body. By expert, I don't mean thinking of a dozen questions to ask our dear friend Google. Start with your local library, as there is no need to invest a ton of money in books if you're not sure they're going to be the right ones. Don't get caught up in books promising cures - you just want to know the ins and outs of the illness.
   o What's going on at a physiological level, and why?
   o What are the side effects of certain medication and how exactly do they work?
   o Learn about possible treatments, both in the eastern and western medical worlds. Jot down the pros and cons of these approaches.

---

[6] Hanger is very real. 3:00 pm is my hangry time of the day. Always.

→ **Slow Down:** You can't become more aware of your body when your calendar runs your life and you survive with a "never-enough-hours-in-the-day" life motto. If you start taking time out of your day to spend just relaxing, you'll start to notice some of the aches and pains your body is experiencing. Then you can ask yourself where that hurt is coming from (whether it's physical or emotional) and start to take the steps towards healing.

→ **Jot Journal:** Don't bring out the fancy leather bound notebook for this part. You need a cheap old 50 cent scribbler from the dollar store. Start the practice of writing down pains when you feel them. Chronic pain? Jot down the highs and lows. When is it keeping you up at night? When do you feel a slight reprieve from that pain? If headaches are plaguing you, start jotting down the days and times that you're noticing them. Do you get a lot of muscle cramps? Jot those down too.

→ **Practice the Pause:** It's natural to want an immediate fix to pain, but numbing discomfort by always reaching for that over-the-counter pain relief is a slippery slope to find yourself on. When that small fix stops working, it's far too easy to move on to other forms of numbing – alcohol, drugs, emotional bingeing on food, or other forms of self-inflicted pain. Instead, practice the Pause. When you feel that headache coming on, start asking questions. Have you been drinking enough water lately? Have you had a proper, nutritious meal? Then scan your body. Is this a tension headache - do you feel it across your shoulders as well? Can you try a relaxation technique in response? Even a short walk outside, or a quick shower if you're at home, can do wonders in relieving some of that tension and helping your headache go away.

→ **Body Scan:** Deepen that awareness of all of the symptoms and signals your body is sending you. The easiest process to follow is to find a comfortable spot to sit or lay down, and then slowly bring awareness to each area of your body, starting at your toes and working your way up to your head. Bring awareness? Sounds so vague, right? I imagine a small flashlight shining on each area as I pause. During that pause I notice any sensations - do I feel any pain? Is that area tight or loose? Cool or warm? That's it. Just notice. Don't analyze. Don't start worrying or comparing. Just notice *what* you feel and *where* you feel it. Then jot it down in your Jot Journal.

"Symptoms are not enemies to be destroyed, but sacred messengers who encourage us to take better care of ourselves."
~ *Unknown* ~

Slowing down and taking time for myself have been the two key ingredients in learning how to tune into my body. I began healing a lot of emotional and physical pain that had been present for a long time, when I stopped numbing and ignoring what my body was trying to tell me.

Your body is a miracle. It really is. It has the innate ability to help you heal, but only if you can slow down and really listen.

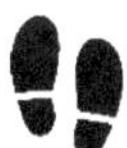 Your Next Steps:

→ Visit the library and check out a book or two on the illness or challenges you're facing. Remember Google is not your friend here.

→ Find a journal to use for your Jot Journal and start writing down the simple things you notice in your body throughout the course of a day, making note of the day and time. Over time, patterns will emerge and you will gain insight into possible causes.

→ Take some time each day to slow down and pause. Find some quiet and just sit. Practice scanning down your body and noticing different things you feel, both good and bad. Use your Jot Journal to make a note about these things too.

"Realize that this very body we have, that's sitting right here right now, with its aches and its pleasures, is exactly what we need to be fully human, fully awake, fully alive."
~ Pema Chodron ~

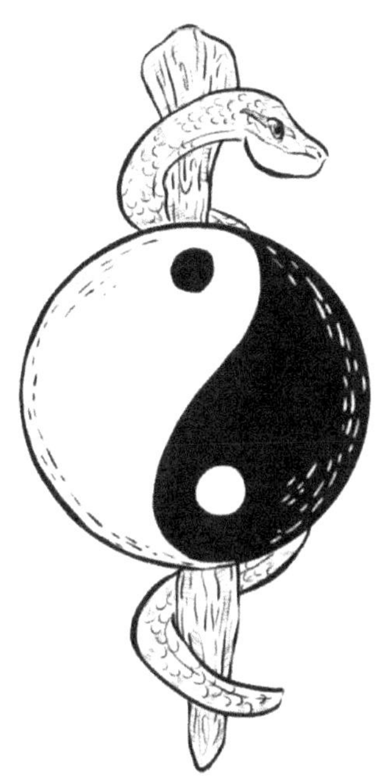

Build Your Health Posse

"A healer is not someone that you go to for healing. A healer is someone that triggers within you, your own ability to heal yourself."
~ *Unknown* ~

I started off building my health "team" with a mix of medical practitioners, spiritual healers and therapists of all different types. And I called it my health team for the longest time but it felt too formal and boring.

So my health posse was born.

> **Posse:** *noun* (pos-se) A group of people who have come together for the same purpose.

Yup, that sounds better. And it gives me the feeling of cohesiveness from this hodge podge collection of doctors and healers that I've found - they all have a common purpose and that is to help me find my path towards healing and better health.

To all of you suffering from illness, this is really important... and to all of you that are as healthy as a horse this is still really important. Building a relationship with your family doctor, and incorporating a variety of other healers into that posse will only bring good things your way, I promise.

As I found the right doctors and healers for my journey, I realized how perfectly Western (modern) medicine and Eastern (complementary) medicine can fit together. Like peanut butter and jelly. I believe that in an ideal world, your healing ability multiplies when you mix these two modes of medicine together.

"Let's build wellness, rather than treating disease."
~ Bruce Daggy ~

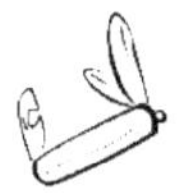 ## *Your Tools:*

→ **An Open Mind:** That's it. You just need to be open to trying as many different forms of healing as necessary to find something that clicks for you.

Your tool is simple, so let's dig into the various options you have at your disposal for continuing on your healing journey.

Family Doctor

You have one, right? If not, I think we can agree on what step one will be. How is your relationship with your doctor? Different people have different needs. While some people value top-notch bedside manner above all else, others wish their doctors were up-to-date on all of the newest studies regarding their illness. There are others who want a well balanced mix of both of those ideals.

The most important thing is that you develop an open and honest relationship with your doctor, where you feel comfortable discussing all aspects of your disease or anything you're experiencing. This sometimes just takes time, but I can tell you with all honesty that I have no issues at this point bringing up poop, the consistency of bowel movements, and how my menstrual cycle is doing. I discuss all of this with my male GP, who doesn't give off the warm and fuzzy vibe, but is extremely knowledgeable and has an insatiable appetite for new knowledge, new studies, and discovering the answer to any problem presented to him.

Massage Therapy

This one is hands down my favourite. The benefits are huge and it's amazing as both a therapeutic and preventative approach to healing. Massage can help reduce or eliminate pain, improve circulation and joint mobility, and help with lymphatic drainage. Massage therapy has also been proven to improve sleep, relieve headaches, and boost immune systems. My husband and I love going for couples massages. Life can be hectic, so when we intentionally take the time to relax and unwind together, it feels like we're benefiting our bodies and our marriage all at the same time.

Physiotherapy

Often doctors will refer their patients to physiotherapists if they believe the service may be beneficial to the patient's healing. However, I sought out my pelvic physiotherapist on my own to help recover from difficulties I was having post-surgery. With visits every 6-8 weeks, my physiotherapist has helped me gain significant momentum with my healing this past year. Like many other forms of healing, physiotherapy addresses the underlying causes and not just the symptoms. I've experienced substantial pain relief, a huge increase in confidence, and the ability to fully function again in areas that were extremely difficult, embarrassing, and causing stress in my life.

Naturopath

This form of complementary medicine is near and dear to my heart because I find that it's the perfect blend of science and nature. Naturopathy digs into addressing the root cause of the illness or disease, rather than just suppressing the symptoms. Doctors trained in naturopathy have a balanced knowledge of conventional medical sciences and natural remedies. They treat the whole person - body, mind, heart, and soul - with an approach that is based on educating and empowering the patient. "Teach, rather than treat" is the main goal. I have been so grateful for the education that I've gained through visits with my naturopath, and the support I've received in believing that my body has the power to heal itself if given the right environment and support system.

Acupuncture

I can be honest and say that I haven't explored this medium very much at all, but I know so many people that have seen the huge benefits found with acupuncture. It is a form of energy healing - designed to release stuck energies and restore balance, facilitating your body's natural ability to heal itself. This branch of medicine has been around for over 2,500 years - making it difficult to discount its healing capabilities. Just like naturopathy, there is no "one size fits all" approach - each patient is treated uniquely, regardless of the disease or other symptoms they might present.

Tapping

This is another form of energy healing that utilizes the body's energy meridian points to literally "tap" into the body's natural ability to heal itself. You don't need to visit a specialist or take special training. A quick search online will lead you to some reputable sources of information to learn how to try this technique out in the comfort of your own home. By tapping your fingers in a sequence through 12 different areas of your body, you help push out the negative energy that is preventing your body from healing, restoring the overall energy balance to a more natural state.

Reiki & Other Energy Healing

One of the largest benefits of energy healing is its ability to promote rest and relaxation, which in turn reduces stress levels in the mind and body. This can trigger our body's natural ability to heal when our negative energy levels have been drastically reduced. Reiki was so foreign to me in the beginning that I was hesitant to try it. Yet it's the least invasive form of healing that I've ever experienced, and the most relaxing and rejuvenating. I find it hard to describe what reiki is, so I'm going to turn to this Mind Body Green article in which reiki practitioner Corinne Feinberg describes it perfectly: "Reiki energy flows where it is most needed to balance and restore anything that is not in harmony within a person's being — physically, mentally, emotionally, and spiritually — and heals parts where life force energy has been affected".

"If you think the pursuit of good health is expensive
and time consuming, try illness."
~ Lee Swanson ~

 **Inspired By...**

Nicole Schmitt of Elle Physiotherapy & Pelvic Health (Red Deer, AB): This incredible woman has facilitated so much of my healing this past year. It turns out that decades of inflammation, two abdominal surgeries, and two pregnancies have really messed with my insides. Go figure? Nicole is full of compassion and is a fountain of knowledge – she teaches me about what exactly is going on inside of my body as she helps me resolve the pain and discomfort that used to be constant. I have learned a boatload about myself and the inner workings of my body this year. I leave every appointment with my body, mind, and heart feeling refreshed and taken care of.

Amanda Joy of Amanda Joy Spiritual Healing (Rocky Mountain House, AB): I attended one of Amanda's yoga retreats in 2016 and I hold her solely responsible for awakening a part of my soul that had been sitting on the sidelines for years. She is an incredible yoga and meditation teacher, but what I am forever grateful for, is the emotional and spiritual healing that she has initiated and given me space for, through reiki and breath work. I feel so safe, loved, and appreciated in Amanda's presence.

Suzanna & Maureen from Sylvan Lake Steam & Spa (Sylvan Lake, AB) : If either of these ladies left their jobs, my husband and I would be devastated. We try to schedule monthly massage dates, and both of these ladies have found the magic behind using intuition to help guide a massage. Each experience is unique and we always leave there feeling like we received exactly what we needed at that moment in time. The fact that it takes us a good five minutes to come back to reality at the end of the massage is testament to the amazing relaxation that these ladies bring to our lives.

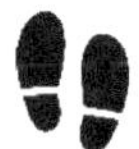 # *Your Next Steps:*

→ Look at your calendar and decide what appointment you should make in the next month. Has it been a while since you've seen your Family Doctor? Do you need to check in? Do you use any of these other healing methods in your life?

"It's more important to understand the imbalances in your body's basic systems and restore balance, rather than name the disease and match the pill to the ill."
~ Mark Hyman ~

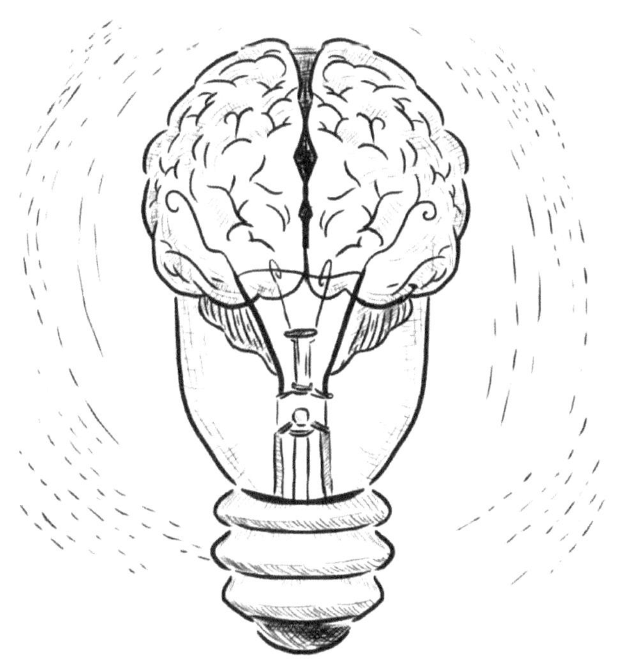

Your Mind

(Section Two)

"The mind is like water. When it is agitated, it becomes difficult to see. But if you allow it to settle, the answer becomes clear."
~ Bil Keane ~

For years, brain fog and fatigue consumed my life. When you're functioning with barely enough energy to complete the most basic of day to day tasks, personal growth and self-improvement get shoved to the back burner pretty easily.

However, after healing my Body, I noticed that my increased energy gave me more motivation, clarity and focus. More energy allowed me to spend time focusing on healing my Mind.

"We cannot become what we need to be,
by remaining what we are."
~ Max DePree ~

Taking care of your intellectual health can be challenging when you are constantly surrounded by clutter and distractions. Our world is bursting at the seams with information overload. Remember the good old days where we only had one place to find the answer to a question like "what's the capital of Switzerland?" We would pull a dusty encyclopedia off the shelf and look it up.

Now we turn to the internet and not only find the answer to our question, but we see 27 advertisements that have been personally fed to us based on our most recent internet searches, over 1,000 results to our Switzerland query, and 52 sparkly squirrels to distract us along the way.

Left to its own devices, it is a recipe for disaster. But you can turn it into a recipe for amazingness if you keep our mantra front and center: **Keep it Simple.**

I learned to embrace these truths about intellectual health in order to finally become unstuck:

- o I will choose to have an open mind, wanting to grow and become the best version of myself.
- o I am in charge of my environment, my time, and the amount of chaos I allow into my life.
- o I will find a passion that makes me come alive and I will shine.

"Don't fear failure. Fear being in the exact
same place next year as you are today."
~ *Unknown* ~

This section is about taking the energy you gain from healing your Body, and using it to take charge of your life with healing your Mind. When you fully take ownership of your life and choose to become the best version of yourself, the empowerment felt is amazing. Healing your Mind is a huge step forward to finding your healthiest, happiest self.

What are you going to work on in this section?

Your Brain Needs Fuel Too - Your Mind needs the right type of energy-boosting fuel, just like your Body does. Focus more on personal development and self-growth.
The Stress of Stuff - Our lives are more cluttered than ever before. Declutter the junk (in your home, your calendar, and your to-do lists) so that you can appreciate the things you love.
Boss of the Clock - Who's in charge of your time? It's you. Only you. Mastering your days, weeks, months, and years is easier than you think.
Find Your Drumbeat - There are natural rhythms in your life, and learning to identify them will help you gain more clarity and focus.
Do What You Love - Passions are important. They increase your desire to learn and grow in an area that ignites the fire in your soul.

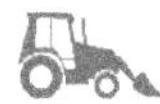

Bring Out the Backhoe...

Essentialism: I believe that after reading (or listening to - the audiobook is fantastic) *Essentialism: The Disciplined Pursuit of Less,* you will start to question all of the "busy work" in your life. You will begin to realize how cluttered and chaotic your life has become, without you even realizing it. It's alarming how the world keeps pushing us to do more, have more, buy more, and be more all of the time. Greg McKeown shares his experiences and insights into why we should do less, but do it better to become the best version of ourselves and live a life true to our values. Directly from his website, this is the best summary out there:
"It's about challenging the core assumption of 'we can have it all' and 'I have to do everything' and replacing it with the pursuit of 'the right thing, in the right way, at the right time'."

The STEP Program by April & Eric Perry: This inspirational couple run a program based off of the idea of "essentialism" (with both a free component and a paid deeper dive into the material). They have taught me how to use a simple process and regular reviews of my projects and tasks to clear the clutter out of my life. I have confidently moved from having overwhelming piles of "stuff" and mile long to-do lists, to a life that has more margin, more clarity, and more stuff getting done. It's just that simple. I would highly recommend checking out their free training at **www.learndobecome.com/stepprogram** to see if it's something that would benefit you.

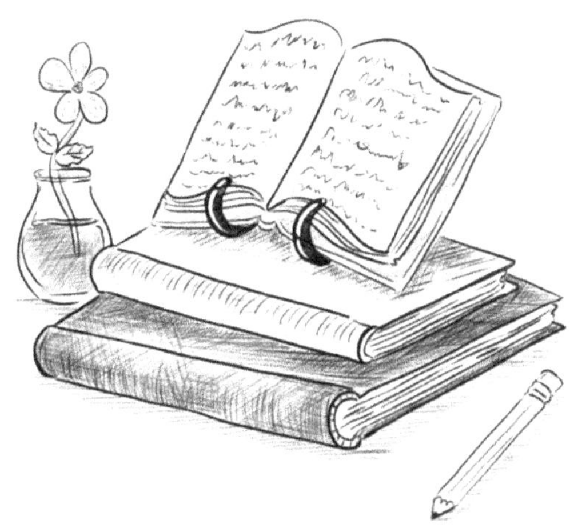

Your Brain Needs Fuel Too

"Reading is to the mind,
what exercise is to the body."
~ Joseph Addison ~

Here's an honest truth from my lonely childhood days: my best friends were Kristy, Claudia, Mary-Anne, and Stacey from the Babysitter's Club. My introverted, mortified-to-talk-to-others self actually loved it though, so looking back I wouldn't have changed that for the world.

Books continued to offer an escape as the years went by. As illness often left me bed and toilet-bound, and fatigue offered me very few functional brain cells to digest new reading material, J.K. Rowling became my knight[7] in shining armour. I read and re-read the Harry Potter series both because the story was fascinating, and because I could escape to a magical world that became familiar over time. The characters and plot lines became a constant while life was continuously unpredictable.

I have also loved devouring books as a form of learning and helping myself grow. Some of the most brilliant minds have shared their discoveries and knowledge with us through the form of books. Isn't it amazing that we can access that knowledge for free through a local library?

Yet it's not quite that simple, is it? I can honestly tell you that I've spent more of the past decade making lists of books I want to read than actually reading them. For years, I have wondered where people actually found the time to pick up a book in their busy lives. In those same years, I spent a ridiculous amount of time playing addictive games on my phone and mindlessly scrolling social media. The answer should have been obvious.

"One must always be careful of books and what is inside them, for words have the power to change us."
~ Cassandra Clare ~

Moving from brain-numbing activities (like wasted time on my phone) to brain-boosting activities (like reading books or listening to audiobooks and podcasts), is hands down one of the best changes I have made on my healing journey. As my mind

[7] Girls can be knights too, right?

became more alive, my focus sharpened and I started having fewer episodes of brain fog taking over.

Beyond focus and clarity, I've grown and developed a lot as a person in the past three years. I'd be bold enough to say that I've grown more intellectually in three years, than in the 15 years before that.[8] Think about the wealth of knowledge that's out there. Books are a gateway into the minds and lives of the most successful and knowledgeable people out there - you can learn and grow so much from them.

In fact, it's not a secret. Many extremely successful people - such as Warren Buffet, Bill Gates, Oprah Winfrey, and Elon Musk - have serious reading habits. They believe in the power of gaining insight and knowledge from the ambitions, mistakes, and successes of people who walked the path before them.

As you embrace the importance of physical exercise and proper nutrition for your body, the next step is to appreciate how your brain needs the right exercise and fuel as well. Reading helps counteract the amount of junk your mind encounters daily by improving your attention span while boosting your memory and overall brain function.

Making reading a priority in my life took a few tweaks and some effort on my part, but now it's a regular part of my routine. Here's what worked for me:

- o Valuing small chunks of time. As lovely as it is to curl up with a good book for an hour in a comfy chair, I keep a book with me to read during all of those times when I'm stuck waiting (in the doctor's office, at my kid's school, etc.)
- o Switching up genres. I like to have both a fiction book (reading for fun) and a non-fiction/personal development book (reading for growth) going at the same time.
- o I also switch it up between e-books on my phone and the good ol' fashioned paperbacks. Adding audiobooks to that arsenal was a fun discovery as I love listening to them while I'm driving.

[8] Which includes 5 years of university and a $50,000 student loan. Stay in school folks, this isn't a cautionary tale - it's just to show you that learning doesn't stop there.

*"Reading forces you to be quiet in a world
that no longer makes place for that."*
~ John Green ~

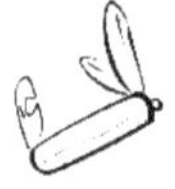 *Your Tools:*

→ **Library Membership:** This is a no-brainer. They're free or ridiculously inexpensive (depending on where you live). The small investment will give you access to thousands of books for free.[9]

→ **Goodreads:** I love this website. It's where I keep track of all the books I want to read, and everything I've read (including a short review when I find the time). But best of all, it's where I get some awesome recommendations based on books I've read or interests I have. When you don't know where to start, or what to read next, this is an amazing tool.

→ **Podcasts:** I'm a humongous fan of audiobooks, but the honest truth is that they are expensive. You can use a free streaming service through your local library, (like Hoopla or Overdrive), but the options of books on those services are usually somewhat limited. The best workaround I've found is turning to podcasts. Most of my favourite non-fiction authors have their own podcasts as well. So I turn to Google Play or Podcast Addict for Android (I hear iTunes and Overcast are the best choices for iPhones) and I listen to some really amazing content. This is perfect for in the car, folding laundry, or going for walks.

→ **Just Doing It:** Little by little, when you find the pockets of

---

[9] Unless you accrue $100 in overdue fines. That's not cool. Not that I would know *anything* about that...

time, read. It's as simple as that.

"The greatest gift is the passion for reading. It is cheap, it consoles, it excites, it gives you knowledge of the world and experience of a wide kind. It is a moral illumination."
~ *Elizabeth Hardwick* ~

 **Inspired By...**

Anne Bogel from Modern Mrs. Darcy: One day I was searching the internet for the world's best homemade latte recipe, and I stumbled upon this website. Not only did I learn how to make a fancy latte without an espresso machine, but I found a goldmine of reading resources. Anne taught me how to make reading a priority and fit time for it throughout the course of my day. I'm still an avid fan - and I visit her blog regularly for advice on books to add to my list. She also has a podcast, *What Should I Read Next,* which is a regular on my playlist. She is 100% to blame for the fact that my Books To Read list is seven miles long. And, she's recently written an amazing book *Reading People*, which is easily on my Top 10 Books of 2017. Needless to say, I'm a super fan.

My Top Five Podcasts:
I'm a podcast addict. These little snippets of useful, insightful information given in 20-60 minute doses are perfect for those shorter drives in the car, or background listening while I'm doing something that doesn't require too much attention. I have gained invaluable knowledge through listening to my favourite authors and speakers share their wisdom and experiences in these podcasts. My top 5 in random order are:
  - *School of Greatness* with Lewis Howes
  - *Happier* with Gretchen Rubin & Elizabeth Kraft

> o   *The Simple Show* with Tsh Oxenreider and multiple
>   co-hosts
> o   *Goal Digger Podcast* with Jenna Kutcher
> o   *The Next Right Thing* with Emily P. Freeman

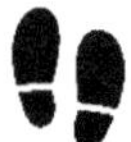 Your Next Steps:

→   Make your **Books To Read** list.

→   Head out to your local library and grab a book today to get
    started. If you're like me, take a look at your bookshelf and
    choose the dustiest book to read next.

→   If you struggle at reading, or it's just not your thing, give
    audiobooks or podcasts a try.

"Books give a soul to the universe, wings to the mind,
flight to the imagination, and life to everything."
~ *Plato* ~

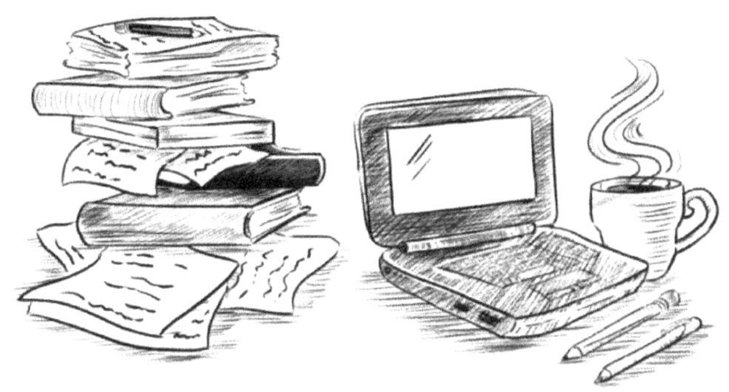

The Stress of Stuff

"Clutter is not just stuff on your floor - it's anything that stands between you and the life you want to be living."
~ Peter Walsh ~

I come from a family of "collectors". From the house I grew up in, to the homes of my grandparents, aunts and uncles, siblings and cousins - most have shelves lined with some of the most interesting trinkets and doo-dads, souvenirs and artifacts.

The truth is that I find it fascinating in other people's homes. Yet in my own, too much stuff - whether on our shelves, in the drawers, or hanging in a closet - gives me anxiety and overwhelms me to my core.

For the past ten years, I've listened to loved ones poke jabs at me about how organized I always was. These were loving jabs, they really were, yet they made me constantly question why I needed the organization so badly. It honestly wasn't for esthetics. I can find homes filled with lots of stuff to be completely charming and cute. It wasn't even because I liked being able to find things, although that's a happy side benefit for sure.

Then I read something that clicked:

"Outer order contributes to inner calm."
~ Gretchen Rubin ~

The author, Gretchen Rubin, talks about how having a crowded coat closet or an overflowing inbox are realistically such trivial matters, yet they tend to weigh us down. She believes that when we feel in control of our stuff, we feel more in control of ourselves and the rest of our lives.

That's it in a nutshell, and it spoke directly to me. All of the external and internal challenges I was facing, whether they were health or grief related, left me feeling out of control in so many areas of my life. I couldn't predict when a flare-up or intestinal blockage was going to happen, and I couldn't predict when I would feel so consumed by grief that I didn't want to get out of bed.

Yet, if my surroundings were in a state of control rather than chaos, that sense of control left me feeling energetic and motivated rather than depressed and depleted.

I've learned that I function at my best (and with drastically reduced amounts of stress and anxiety in my daily life) if I can declutter these three areas: my mind, my time, and my home.

When you apply the **Keep it Simple** approach to your mind, your time, and your home, you can simplify your life to the point where the excess clutter is controlled and you can start living the life you want to live.

"Clutter is nothing more than postponed decisions..."
~ Barbara Hemphill ~

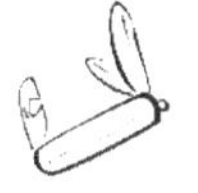 ## Your Tools:

→ **Brain Dump:** We all have these spider-webs of to-dos, reminders, tasks, and ideas that are swirling around in our heads, taking up valuable space and wasting precious time. To do a Brain Dump, sit down with a pen and piece of paper. Now start jotting down everything that you need and want to get done. Things like:
  o   Appointments that need to be made
  o   Errands you need to run
  o   Projects you want to start
  o   Projects you need to finish
  o   Birthday presents to be purchased
  o   A dream or goal that you wish for, ten years from now
The important part here is that it needs to be anything and everything that is taking up space in your Mind.[10]
Know that above all, it is completely okay (and even a really good thing) if your list is 5 pages long. It often is in the beginning. You'll learn how to filter and organize this list later. Right now, just get it out of your brain.

---

[10] Emotions, pet peeves, and soul searching questions included

→ **Purge the Physical Stuff:** This gets a little tricky because there is no one-size-fits-all approach. Two of the best approaches are going room-by-room or category by category (clothing, media, paperwork, etc.)
   o Decide what is important, and keep that stuff. Display it if you can, or store it in keepsake containers that you pull out once in a while to re-live happy memories.
   o Get rid of what is causing you any source of stress. As you go through your house, you'll know what this is. If your gut reaction is "ugh, I'll deal with that later" - chances are that object is a source of stress that you need to deal with now.

→ **Get Your Time Back:** If you spend more time away from home than at home, do a major review of your calendar. If you feel over scheduled in any way, commit to removing something from that schedule. You can, even though I know it can be a challenge.
   o **Balance home days with away days.** Rather than running out to do errands every day of the week, can you lump a bunch of them together? The same goes for activities that need to happen at home (like laundry, meal prep, and house projects). Lump those activities together so you get more done in a single stretch of time.
   o **Define what "priority" means to you and your family.** There's no right answer, and it's different for everyone. If your family's priority is to spend more time together, then cut out some of the extra-curricular activities from your life. Believe it or not, kids grow up completely well balanced without filling their lives with activities. However, if your family's priority is to pursue your passions and you have kids that are extremely passionate about a certain activity, then cut out some other "fillers" and make the important things stand out above all else in your calendar.

"What if we stopped celebrating being busy as a measurement of importance? What if instead we celebrated how much time we had spent listening, pondering, meditating, and enjoying time with the most important people in our lives?"
~ Greg McKeown ~

The most welcome side effect of this whole decluttering plan is the elimination of decision fatigue.

- o With my mind dumped out on paper, it's easier for me to see what things absolutely need to get done and start crossing them off of the overflowing to-do list.
- o With less in my closet, it's painless for me to decide what to wear in the mornings.
- o With less clutter lying around, a simple house tidy is all that is needed.
- o With a clearcr view of my calendar, it's simple for me to plan coffee dates with friends, connect with my husband and kids, and find downtime for doing things I love to do.

More than anything though, finding my solution to the Stress of Stuff in my life freed me from feelings of overwhelm and anxiety. That is definitely worth its weight in gold.

 **Inspired By...**

Tsh Oxenreider: She has been an important mentor of mine over the years. I love her blog, her podcast, and all of her books. She's the founder of *The Art of Simple,* a blog about what simple living means to different people, and I have been following along on her journey for many, many years. I love how she stresses that there is no such thing as a one-size fits all approach to simple living.

Marie Kondo: Founder of the KonMari method and author of two decluttering books - *The Life Changing Magic of Tidying Up* and *Spark Joy.* Her method of keeping only the things that "spark joy" in your home, can be a somewhat controversial topic as a lot of people like to point out that their kitchen whisk or tube of deodorant do not, in fact, spark joy. Yet, her key philosophy around making our homes a place that inspire and reflect our values, rather than a dumping ground for more and more stuff, rings loud and true.

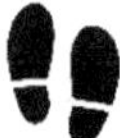 # Your Next Steps:

→ Do an initial Brain Dump. Then practice the habit of doing mini dumps before you go to bed at night. Get that unnecessary clutter out of your Mind.

→ Collect your first box of donations from your house. Put the box directly into your car and get it to the second-hand store as soon as possible. Good job! Now start collecting your second box.

→ Look at your calendar. What unnecessary event or activity can you eliminate? Do this regularly, either weekly or even monthly.

"What I know for sure is that when you declutter - whether it's in your home, your head, or your heart - it is astounding what will flow into that space that will enrich you, your life, and your family."
~ *Peter Walsh* ~

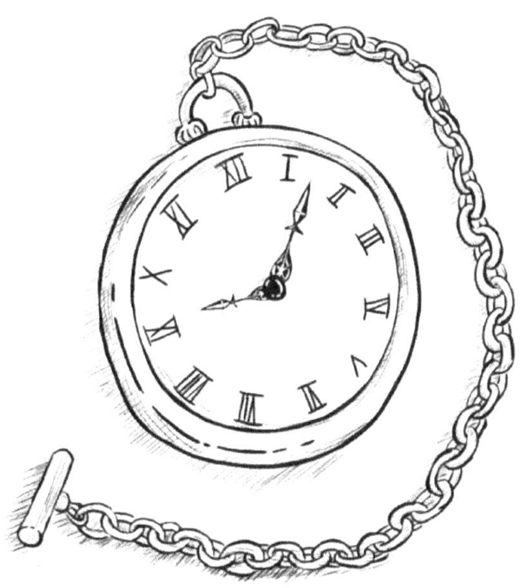

Boss of the Clock

"You are who you essentially create yourself
to be and all that occurs in your life is the
result of your own making."
~ Stephen Richards ~

Two years ago I made one of the biggest changes that helped me stop just drifting through my days. I became the CEO of my life.

That's right. I even conjure up the image of myself sitting behind a fancy desk in my plush executive office chair, making the decisions about how my day, week, and year need to look in order to be the most successful version of myself that I can be. Visuals are important people.

It sure took a while to make that realization though - to fully understand that I was the only one who could plan my days and life in a way that made me feel less crazy and overwhelmed.

I was a pro at just letting my days happen. However they happened. I'd wake up to kids pulling me out of bed and I would go through all of the motions that needed to be done. Stress would pile higher on my shoulders as more things jumped on my to-do list than got crossed off. I would ping pong back and forth between tasks, until late in the evening when I would crash into bed and sleep restlessly until the next morning when it happened all over again.

I was stuck in my own Groundhog Day hell.

"The bad news is - time flies.
The good news is - you're the pilot."
~ Michael Altshuler ~

The road to CEO was a little bumpy. I discovered some excellent mentors – various authors of books on time management who taught me how to take control of my time. They helped me find the right mindset and develop an understanding that I was in charge of my days and my time, and I could waste them or become more successful, the choice was mine. But putting those ideas into practice was a little more complicated than I realized.

I was so bogged down with fatigue that I had no idea where to start. My motivation was high, but the fatigue kept winning the battle every day. I didn't know what to do.

Then, one day I visited my soul-sister. My kindred spirit who has the same disease, has underwent the same surgeries, and laughs and cries with me through the same struggles.

Paula: "You should think about seeing an occupational therapist. I learned a lot from mine."

Me: "That's an awesome suggestion." *(Inner voice: "I think I need a little more than an adjustment to my office chair.")* [11]

Her suggestion played over and over in my head enough times that I eventually booked an appointment. I was hooked after the initial consult. This amazing therapist taught me a ton about how to manage my time and stresses in life. Here's the conversation that led to my breakthrough:

Me: "I just feel overwhelmed... like... all of the time."

Therapist: "What parts of your life are overwhelming?"

Me: "Being a mom, taking care of the kids and the house, the simplest day-to-day stuff like laundry, being there for my husband when I don't even have the energy to have a shower most days..." *(I felt embarrassed and ashamed saying any of this out loud. I thought it made me sound so weak and incapable.)*

Therapist: "What if you took all of those balls that you're juggling and just tried to focus on one at a time?"

Me: "Sounds great." *(Inner voice: "Um right, don't you get it? I have to do ALL OF THE THINGS!")*

She gave me an exercise. To make a list of all of my roles (Mom, Wife, Me, Volunteer, etc.) and my responsibilities for each. I was the reluctant student who couldn't see how this was going to help me actually get stuff done, but I did it anyways.

This exercise taught me the art of Time Blocking. I was instructed to take each of my roles and assign them a chunk of time throughout the day, doing tasks related to that particular role during that block of time. If you think back to generations before us, they were experts at this - they wouldn't have interrupted their cow milking routine 12 different times to do

---

[11] Oh, how naïve and closed-minded once again...

other random, minor tasks. Somewhere along the line though, we've lost touch with this.

"People often complain about lack of time
when the lack of direction is the real problem."
~ Zig Ziglar ~

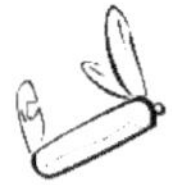 ## Your Tools:

→ **Identify Your Roles:** What hats do you wear throughout the week? List all of them: Mom/Dad, Employee, Home-Keeper[12], Volunteer, Wife/Husband, Friend, Girlfriend/Boyfriend. Only list the ones that apply to you. And most importantly don't forget Me. You are your most important role and taking Me Time to take care of yourself is often the most important change you can make in your life.

→ **Know Your Responsibilities:** Those hats come with jobs for each. It helps to know everything you do in your various roles, so tackling a specialized brain dump for each is extremely useful. Think about all of the tasks that you do daily, weekly, monthly, and annually.

→ **Build Time Blocks into Your Days:** Take a blank sheet of paper with the days of the week written at the top. Now start scheduling your roles into your schedule. Put in the non-negotiables first. If you work from 8-4 every weekday, make sure that time is blocked off. If you get an hour off at lunch and you can use that time for connecting with friends or exercising (Me Time), put those blocks into your schedule. Is Saturday morning a good time to take care of your home? Put that block of time into the schedule.

---

[12] Easier than listing out chef, cleaner, chauffeur, repairman, etc.

→ **Get Rid of the Squirrels:** The squirrels in our life are all of the distractions that pop up and throw us off track. They cause us to endlessly spin on a hamster wheel that looks something like this:

> *Tidy, tidy, tidy... "Oh, I have to reply to that email"... sit down at computer to type out email. "And that soccer registration is due tomorrow". Move to soccer page and fill out form. "Crap, where are those soccer shin pads?"... Head downstairs to search... "Wow, when's the last time these stairs were vacuumed?"... Drags out vacuum...*

One simple change is to turn off most notifications on your phone. There was no real reason why I needed to be alerted with every single email that came in, not to mention every Facebook notification. I am much less distracted now that I don't hear beeps and buzzes all day long. Instead I plan a couple of times a day where I check in with email and social media, but on my time and not at the drop of a hat.

→ **Make Me Time a Priority:** This is the easiest one to forget or sweep under the rug. However, when Me Time becomes more of a priority, it actually becomes way easier to keep your focus on all of the other things.

> "The key is not to prioritize what's on your schedule,
> but to schedule your priorities."
> ~ Stephen Covey ~

Please note however, that Time Blocking never, ever looks perfect. My scheduled House Time where I do dinner prep and laundry will inevitably get interrupted with a dozen requests, questions, and world-ending catastrophes from the kids. My Kid Time will get stopped short when the phone rings. But overall there is way less ping-ponging back and forth between all of my tasks.

Maybe it didn't look perfect, but my days flowed with more ease and I felt a weight lift off of my shoulders. Time was no longer the boss of me because I controlled the hours of my days. Here's the truth of adulting: no one else is going to do that for you.

 **Inspired By...**

Getting Things Done by **David Allen:** Following the advice in this book has been a game changer for me. The author, David Allen, offers a very easy to follow, step-by-step approach to organizing your ideas, your schedule, and your to-do's in a way that makes everything more manageable. His subtitle sums up the value I get from this system: "the art of stress-free productivity" - it truly is an art, which makes me love it even more. And Mr. Allen, you had me at "stress-free".

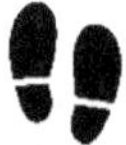 *Your Next Steps:*

→ Write out your Roles (all of the hats you wear).

→ Brain dump the Responsibilities (tasks) for each hat, just for the next week.

→ Look at your calendar, add those jobs into your week in time blocks (put similar tasks together to avoid ping-ponging back and forth).

"Either you run the day, or the day runs you."
~ Jim Rohn ~

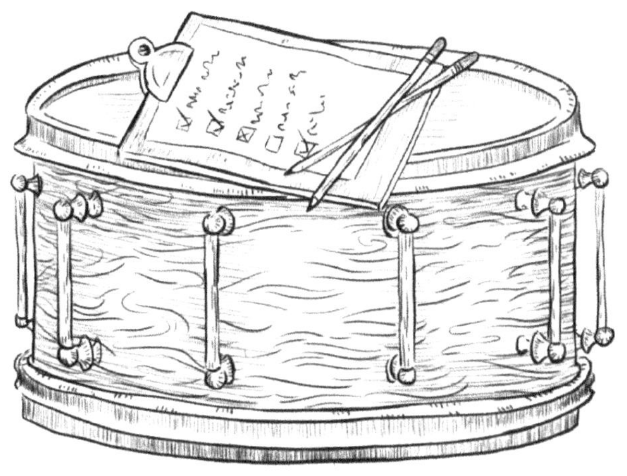

Find Your Drumbeat

"We are what we repeatedly do.
Excellence then, is not an act but a habit."
~ Aristotle ~

How could I be busy all day long, never taking a minute to just sit and relax, and **still** there are the same 12 things on my to-do list as there were first thing this morning?

I lived this life for years. Running from day to day getting nothing accomplished on my list, but still doing 39 random things. My mornings were spent scrambling to get us ready for the day and cleaning up the kitchen from the night before. My afternoons were spent hustling through all of the tasks that weren't done yesterday or last week. Then my evenings were spent rushing to figure out what we were eating for supper and catching up with kids' homework and activities.

The end of the day would come and I would review the mental checklist of everything that I had wanted to get done that day. Not even the have-to stuff, but my want-to list. And frustration would flood over me as I sat there baffled as to how I could ever make it work.

I wanted to:
- o   Exercise
- o   Plan & prep for healthy meals
- o   Meditate
- o   Commit to a before-bed routine so that I achieved better sleep
- o   Read more books
- o   Spend quality time with friends & family
- o   Squeeze in more one-on-one time with my husband and kids

There wasn't "save the dolphins" or "end world hunger" on that list. It should have been easier to make it happen.

"Success is the sum of small efforts, repeated day in and day out."
~ Robert Collier ~

A disagreement with our tweenager changed all of that. I was frustrated with her because she'd forgot, for the umpteenth time in a row, to put in her retainer that she's supposed to wear every night. She was frustrated with me because once again, I was nagging. A normal parent/kid disagreement ensued that sounded like this:

Mom: "Why do we have to have this conversation every single morning?" *(my voice raising in frustration)* "What are you going to do to change this?"

Tween: "I'm just going to start doing it. I'll just start doing it!"

Mom: "That won't work!" *(my voice still raised)* "Your mind won't know how to 'just start doing something'. You need a plan!"

Pause. Silence from both of us - she wasn't sure why I was suddenly staring into space, and I had realized that I was the pot calling the kettle black.

I needed a plan. And if I could make this happen in my life, I'd be a much better mentor to help our kids develop the habits that they needed in theirs.

"Life is a balance between what we can control and what we cannot.
I am learning to live between effort and surrender."
~ Danielle Orner ~

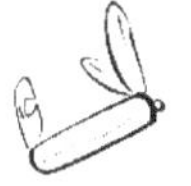 # Your Tools:

→ **Look for Rhythms in your Tasks:** Take your List of Hats & Tasks from the *Boss of the Clock* chapter and start to make lists of your daily, weekly, and monthly rhythms. You'll start to see patterns.

→ **Look for Rhythms in your Life:** We all have seasonal patterns too. There are months or sometimes particular days (for example the anniversary of the death of a loved one) where life starts to feel off-balance. For some people, the holiday season can be stressful and overwhelming. For others, it's getting through the dead of winter in February where anxiety or depression raise their ugly heads. Start paying attention to what those triggers or seasons are in your life. When you know what they are and when they occur, you can begin to discover how you should respond to them.

→ **Start Your Day on Purpose:** Do you feel frazzled when you wake up to kids pulling you out of bed, plummeting you with their list of demands? Things like "I'm hungry", "I lost my blankie!" and "Can you wipe my bum?"[13] Or maybe it's not kids that jumpstart your mornings. Do you enjoy waking up to the alarm, hitting snooze four times, and then rushing through the motions as you get your day started? Doesn't waking up to a cup of fresh coffee and reading a chapter in a good book sound like a better alternative? Learning how to be in control of the first hour of your day is one of the best things you can do. Life starts running much more efficiently.

→ **Win The Day the Night Before:** An awesome morning starts with the night before. I try to win each day by doing a handful of things the night before so that the morning runs smoother, such as:
  o Get everything ready for your morning cup of coffee.
  o Pack lunches the night before - no more flying by the seat of your pants in the morning.
  o Do you exercise first thing? Get your workout clothes and shoes out and ready with your water bottle so that there's no excuses.
  o Do you journal or read first thing? Have those things set out so that you can continue with that intention instead of getting sidetracked with a load of laundry that needs to be folded.
  o Wake up to a clean sink and counters. This is a big one for me. Maybe it isn't for you, but when I wake up in the morning and there are no dishes to catch up on or crap to put away, my morning and rest of the day is much more successful. I'm a stickler about kitchen

---

[13] Oh... the joys of potty training.

cleanup after supper – the whole family pitches in because they love seeing a happy Mommy!

"Your day is pretty much formed by how you spend your first hour. Check your thoughts, attitude, and heart."
~ *Unknown* ~

Learning to move to the rhythm of your life - throughout your days, weeks, and seasons - will bring so much more balance to your entire life.

 **Inspired By…**

Gretchen Rubin: Her book *Better Than Before*, was a game-changer for me. Her strategies for getting started include building healthy habits into our lives and solutions for the roadblocks many of us face. She encourages finding the strategies that work best for us by answering questions along the way to get to know ourselves better. This way, we can tailor our habit forming systems to achieve *our* best results, independent of what works best for others. Her bold claim really is true: "If we change our habits, we change our lives."

Crystal Paine: I have taken two wonderful courses from this mentor of mine – *Makeover Your Mornings* and *Makeover Your Evenings*. Both have helped me manage the beginning and end of my day with routines that change the entire dynamic of our house. When I can stick to these rhythms, our lives feel calmer and our days run much smoother because everyone knows what to expect next. The best part is the importance these rhythms place on doing things to help me take care of myself, not just my family.

> **Kendra Adachi:** Another influential mentor of mine. Her blog and podcast *The Lazy Genius* are both full of advice and actionable tips on how to find the rhythms in your life. Her main goal is to help us "become a genius about the things that matter, and lazy about the things that don't". She wants to help all of us stop trying to do it all, and stop living by a list of "shoulds". She's hilarious, down-to-earth, and her advice in many areas has helped me immensely.

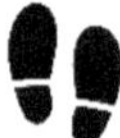 ## Your Next Steps:

→ Schedule Me Time at the beginning of your day. It can be as short as 10 minutes or as long as an hour. Do what works for you, and pick 2-3 things you can do as soon as you wake up that get your day started on the right foot.

→ Make your Win The Day list and start doing those things in the evenings before you get ready for bed. What can you do to make tomorrow run smoother?

→ Other routines and rhythms will follow. Start here for now.

"You'll never change your life until you change something you do daily. The secret of your success is found in your daily routine."
~ John Maxwell ~

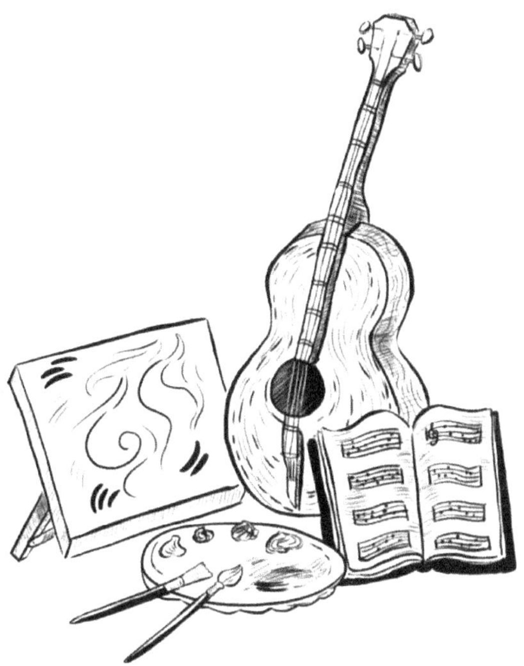

Do What You Love

"Be fearless in the pursuit of
what sets your soul on fire."
~ Unknown ~

Do you have a thing? A thing you do, that while you're doing it, you completely lose track of time and the rest of the world just melts away. We could also call it a "passion", but I happen to love the cozy, comfortable, best friend feeling that comes along with calling it a "thing". I'll probably call it both names.

I was missing a thing for a very long time. Well, not really. It was technically always there and it's been there since I was a little kid... but I ignored it for years.

The biggest hurdle in my way of finding my thing was that I was trying everybody else's passions and interests on for size, thinking that I could just copy and paste. Scrapbooking, sewing, photography, sketching, knitting[14].

For years I didn't pursue a passion, and the truth is that it bothered me a little inside. I witnessed people all around me blossoming and blooming in so many ways as they followed what set their souls on fire.

It was a constant inspiration, and all of these passion-seekers sill inspire me daily. Most members of my family seem to have this knack for discovering something they love to do. Photography, art-making, book-binding, snowboarding, adventure-seeking, blanket-making, computer-coding, running, quilting, welding, gardening, snowmobiling, and the list goes on.

They have all been using their passions as an outlet for creative expression. That's where the magic lies. Snowboarding is definitely not a passion for all of us - for me it's a cold and frustrating way to get physical activity in the wintertime, as I spend more time on my butt than cruising down the hill. But for others, they truly come alive out on that ski hill. You can see it in their photos and you can hear it in their voices as they share their stories. And if you dug a little deeper, and asked them if it brings joy to their lives, the answer would be an emphatic "yes!"

I think that's how you know it's a passion, how you know you've found your 'thing'.

I'm sure you've figured out by now what my thing is, right? You're looking at it. Putting words on paper, through a pen or

---

[14] Does seven loops on a needle count as knitting? Gave up on that one quickly...

the click-clack of a keyboard, that's the passion that could keep me up all night long if I let it. It's what has set my soul on fire and keeps my mind growing and thriving.

"Whatever it is that stirs your soul, listen to that.
Everything else is just noise."
~ Nicole Lyons~

Some people call these hobbies. But there's this poetic side of me that says it's more than just a hobby - it's what makes you come alive inside. It's the thing that you'll find the time to fit into your schedule, above all else.

And for those of us that can't find our passions, what are we doing wrong? Sounds like the common flaw we have is that we're looking too hard. We're expecting our passion to have a particular look or feel, and we observe others, lamenting on the woe of "it must be nice, to have found your passion."

I love the article *Screw Finding Your Passion* written by Mark Manson, He reminds us that as kids we had no issues finding things we loved to do because we were led by our excitement and curiosity, nothing else. He says:

"And if you loved looking for bugs, you just did that. There was no second level analysis of, "Well, is looking for bugs really what I should be doing with my time as a child?
Nobody else wants to look for bugs, does that mean there's something wrong with me? How will looking for bugs affect my future prospects?"
~ Mark Manson ~

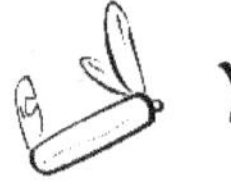 # *Your Tools:*

→ **Open Mindset:** I know people who have said "I'm not a runner, I hate running"... and then they start doing it for another random reason and grow to love it. Your passion might actually be something that surprises you.

→ **Persistence:** If at first you don't succeed, try again. When you're not sure if you've found your thing, you definitely haven't. Keep trying. Over and over again, until you do.

→ **Kill the Comparison Complex:** Remember the phrase "Comparison is the thief of joy"? It so important to remember this as we find the passion that sparks joy inside.

"When you recover or discover something that nourishes your soul and brings you joy, care enough about yourself to make room for it in your life."
~ Unknown ~

Doing something that makes you come alive inside doesn't mean that you need to be the 'best' at. It's the opposite - you do the things you love doing, just because you love them and for the way they make you feel inside.

When you're passionate about something, you're willing to keep learning and growing in that area. In fact, you're excited about becoming better and learning more about the things you love doing. The very act of doing something repeatedly, naturally makes you become increasingly better at it.

Having a passion keeps you grounded and in the present moment. It can be an excellent method of stress relief as it takes your mind off of worrying about the past or future, and more focused on doing something in the right here, right now.

 **Inspired By...**

Paula Timm of Paula Timm Art (Calgary, AB): My dear friend is an art instructor and wellness advocate. She encourages others to find the healing relationship between wellness and creativity and works with the motto: "your creativity is a gift, it can heal, just watch yourself grow." Through facilitating art classes that are based on exploring your creativity and letting it guide you, Paula has helped many others discover the healing powers of igniting that creative spark inside of themselves.

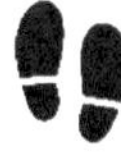 ## Your Next Steps:

→ If you have a passion and you know exactly what it is, keep doing it.

→ If you don't have a passion, make a list of things you'd like to try. Then try them. Repeat until you've found your thing, and then keep doing it.

"Passion is energy. Feel the power that comes
from focusing on what excites you."
~ Oprah Winfrey ~

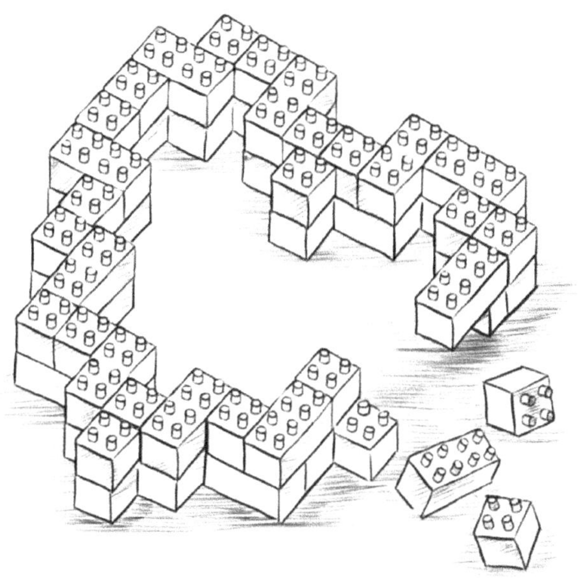

Your Heart

(Section Three)

"And if I asked you to name all of the
things that you love, how long would it take
you to name yourself?"
~ Unknown ~

If your Body is the most vital area you can work on, and your Mind is the most empowering area, then your Heart is definitely the most valuable.

It is also the most overlooked area of the Healing Compass. This is the space where we make the most excuses, where we don't have the right tools, and where we feel shame or disconnection in so many different ways.

"Let's not forget that the little emotions are the great captains of our lives and we obey them without realizing it."
~ Vincent Van Gogh ~

Last year, my five year old son came to me really upset about a Lego creation that had been modified by one of his sisters - something insignificant in my eyes. "No big deal" is the label I put on it, yet he was hysterical, with tears streaming down his cheeks and his voice raised as he gave me his high-pitched version of the events that had transpired. He was devastated - both hurt and angry about this tiny little thing that was monumental in his eyes.

My practical (but lacking compassion) advice for him: "You have to toughen up son. Brush it off. Not the end of the world." I'm sure that I was super "busy" at the time, and dealing with yet another interruption to my day was frustrating.

Every parent out there can relate, right? How many of these world-ending events transpire on a daily basis? And if you don't have kids, how many times has your partner or a friend vented about a personal struggle where your internal reaction was along the lines of, "Are you serious?"?

These emotional breakdowns with kids can be frequent, but this one in particular stuck with me. It was the perfect example of how much I needed to work on understanding and healing my own Heart, so that I could help my kids with theirs. How on earth could I expect my five year old son to know how to handle hurt and disappointment if I was over here failing miserably as well?

"Quick to judge, quick to anger, slow to understand...
prejudice, fear and ignorance walk hand in hand."
~ *Peart* ~

Why is our emotional health so often overlooked and undervalued? How many of us have actually been given the tools or coaching to work on our emotions? Did somebody teach you how to grieve? Have you ever been made fun of for expressing certain emotions in certain ways? On the same token, are you able to effectively teach others how to regulate their emotions, how to respond to stress, or how to grieve?

Society struggles with speaking about emotional health. We're starting to make headway and my heart expands tenfold every time that I see someone speak publicly about their battles with depression, anxiety, grief, or loneliness. But we still have a long way to go.

What are you going to work on in this section?

Medicine for Your Heart: Therapy. It is the best thing that has ever happened for me, yet it's underused in society because of stigma, uncertainty, and shame. Let's change that.
Pen & Paper: You need an outlet for your emotions. By expressing yourself through a creative outlet, you will work through processing emotions, not bottling them.
Connect the Dots: Relationships are key. Connect every single day, in some way.
A New Kind of Self-Care: Learn how to understand yourself, how to love yourself, and how to make time to really take care of yourself.
Finding Dandelions: Embrace the crappy parts of life, so you can truly feel the joy. Sitting in darkness isn't as scary as it sounds, for the light always follows.

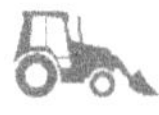

Bring Out the Backhoe...

A Letting it Go Practice: One of my therapists gave me this exercise to do, and now I make it a regular part of my routine whenever my emotional health is feeling out of balance.

First, identify the emotion or feeling that's coming up frequently for you. It could be frustration, sadness, guilt, or overwhelm, to name a few. Now find a good chunk of time - 30 minutes or so where you can write freely, being completely open and vulnerable about everything in your life that's triggering that feeling or emotion. The first time I did this it was about "guilt" and I thought of three things, then called it good. And then I realized that I was being pathetic and closed minded, and went back and bawled my head off as I wrote another 37 things that I felt guilty about. Some felt lame as I was writing them down (ex: "I feel guilty about feeding my kids too much cereal..."). The truth trumps lameness – remember that. Now that you have your list, it's time to let it go. You have a few options:

- o Roll that piece of paper up, find a body of water and let it set sail. There is something extremely cathartic about the healing powers of water and letting your negative thoughts and emotions be cleansed and erased, giving you a clean slate to start from.
- o Find a fireplace or fire pit and set your negative thoughts and emotions on fire. Let them go. Let the flames obliterate and erase every ounce of negativity and give you a clean slate to start from.
- o Take your piece of paper and rip it into tiny shreds, once again, destroying the negative energy and giving you a clean slate to start from.

Such a simple exercise. It's amazing to see the number of feelings and irrational connections we hold on to. Releasing those can help your Heart heal immensely.

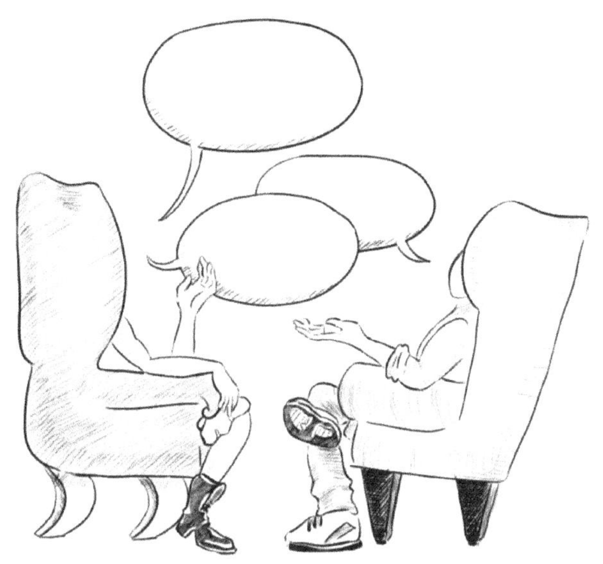

Medicine for Your Heart

"People start to heal the moment
they feel heard."
~ *Cheryl Richardson* ~

We all rely on the little flashing lights on our vehicle's dashboard to let us know when something is wrong and that it's time to get a tune-up from the mechanic. We don't wait for the vehicle to leave us stranded on the side of the road with smoke pouring out from under the hood before we seek help from a car expert.

Yet, we usually ignore the warning signals and signs of distress that our Heart sends our way. We will seek a dentist when we have a toothache, or search for a personal trainer when we want to get fit. But when our Heart is hurting or when we feel overwhelmed with emotion and anxiety - do we jump up to call a therapist to help get our emotional health back on track again?

Chances are unlikely. We'll wait for that total emotional breakdown, the smoke pouring out from our Hearts leaving us at rock bottom, and then maybe we'll find a good therapist to talk to.

"Until you make the unconscious conscious,
it will direct your life and you will call it fate."
~ Carl Jung ~

This past year I had my own emotional breakdown. There were many occasions that had me bawling my head off without a reason why, tense with anger and no justifiable trigger, or consumed with sadness and loneliness even as I was surrounded by the most loving family and friends in the world.

In hindsight, labeling myself as A Wreck would be a serious understatement. Yet, I presented as this happy, cheerful, "always making lemonade out of lemons", strong woman.

Behind the scenes, I was perfecting the art of bottling up emotions. Every negative emotion that came on my radar I would let myself experience for a moment, and then throw a label on it and tuck it away, either with the intention of "dealing with it later" or under the false pretense of "I've dealt with that" when I definitely had not.

"When we deny the story, it defines us. When we own the story,
we can write a brave new ending."
~ Brené Brown ~

Imagine my Heart having an Emotion Room lined with dozens upon dozens of shelves. Over the years, my art of bottling had these shelves overflowing with bottle after bottle of all the feelings. It sure was neat and tidy, with all of them lined up in rows, but these shelves were starting to get a little heavy. And when they collapsed – when all of those bottles came crashing down in this massive wreck on the floor – I was a wreck as well.

I hit rock bottom with my emotional health. When I started to see how negatively it was impacting my marriage and my relationship with my kids, I knew things had to change.

I found a therapist that I connected with, and began learning about tools to heal my Heart. It was a difficult step and it required me to be more open and vulnerable than I was comfortable with at first. Some sessions saw many tears, and others had some breakthroughs, but they all left me feeling like another layer was peeled off and some weight was lifted off my shoulders. I've learned some valuable tools during my time in therapy and I'll share them with you here.

Your Tools:

→ **Wait for 48** (the 24/48 Hour Rule):
When something is a big enough trigger to make me feel angry or hurt, I always try to sit on it for a bit. I define a big trigger as something that causes me to react with frustration or anger, not just something that pushes my buttons. I've learned to wait for 48 hours with all of the big triggers I feel, rather than having that knee-jerk reaction with an over the top response.

When I first feel the hurt creep in, I follow Brené Brown's advice - she says "don't talk, text or type". We can sometimes jump straight into wanting to throw blame at someone else for the hurt or shame we're feeling.

Texting, emailing, or phoning the person I want to toss blame at is never a good idea. Instead, I sit down with my journal and write it out. When I don't feel like writing, I sometimes go for a walk and talk to the trees.[15] Getting words off of my chest in solitude is often the antidote to my negative feelings, and keeps me from bottling them up.

Next, I shift my perspective and put the shoe on the other foot. When I recognize that someone else might be going through their own difficult situation or feelings, the compassion I feel eliminates that initial negative reaction.

→ **The Button Pusher List:**
Chances are there is a theme or pattern to your small emotional triggers. It will help to identify what those button pushers are. Start by making a list of everything that drives you a little bit crazy. By having a list, you can start to see that many of these small triggers are actually within your control. Next, learn some simple coping techniques that will help you stop wasting emotional energy on them.

- **Pause & Breathe:** Eliminate that knee jerk response by taking a pause and thinking about the bigger picture. Ask yourself "will this matter 5 minutes from now? 5 hours from now? 5 days from now?" Don't put a negative reaction out in the world for something that doesn't deserve your emotional energy. Remember, your emotion reservoir is limited - save it for the happiness and joy in your life.

- **Take a Time-Out.** When a simple pause and deep breath isn't enough, remove yourself from the situation for a few minutes. I have Mommy Time Outs - I find them way more effective than sending my kid for a time-out when my buttons get pushed. I can usually gain better

---

[15] I'm not exaggerating – they're amazing listeners

perspective on a situation and respond, rather than react, when I'm ready.

→ **Honour Your Losses:**
Grief is such a difficult emotion to process. Probably because it's more than just an emotion; it feels like a physical force that can take over your whole life. Another challenge is that our western society seems to attach a clock to our grieving experience. As if we should be sad for a bit and then move on. End of story. I've done my fair share of grieving and although I feel supported and understood in the time immediately after losing a loved one, I feel like people look at me questionably when I openly grieve months or years later. After losing my sister, I sought out grief counselling. "Society tells us that the first year is the hardest," my therapist told me, "but the truth is it will be hard on and off for the rest of your life. One of the biggest gifts you can give yourself is to set aside time every day to honor the person you've lost." Now, I honor my dad and sister daily through writing letters, lighting candles, or talking out loud to their spirits. Rituals have a profound effect - doing a simple act of reflection connects our mind, heart, and spirit.

"We repeat what we don't repair."
~ *Christine Langley-Obaugh* ~

Therapy has so many benefits, and if the only thing holding you back is your belief that it's "just not right for you", then maybe that's a topic you could discuss with your therapist. Seriously, it's for everyone. It's like saying "I don't believe in the power of antibiotics to cure an infection." Science can prove otherwise. Same with therapy.

👣 *Your Next Steps:*

If you're ready to take that step, to seek out therapy in one form or another, here are some excellent places to start:

→ **Psychology Today** – www.psychologytoday.com has an amazing "Find A Therapist" section where you can look through their extensive listings for a Therapist, Psychiatrist, Group Support, or Treatment Centres in your area. Their directory encompasses Canada and the United States.

→ **Good Therapy** - www.goodtherapy.org has another extensive directory for therapists across Canada and the United States, with detailed filters to help you narrow down your results.

"Deep in your wounds are seeds, waiting to grow beautiful flowers."
~ Niti Majethia ~

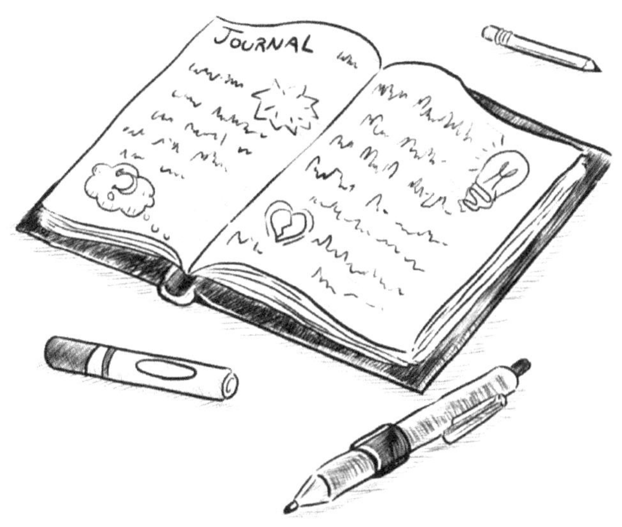

Pen & Paper

"Write about the colour of pain,
and the taste of happiness."
~ Unknown ~

Words have power. You know this. The bully that says mean things can have a detrimental impact on an entire childhood. And those words that lift you up in spirit can be worth their weight in gold.

Before we go a little deeper on why I believe words are so important, let's look at creativity in general as a tool for healing and happiness. It's not all about words and using a pen and paper. There's a bigger picture here that involves engaging in a creative process of some kind, any kind, that helps heal your Heart.

Moving beyond pen and paper, creativity might look like:

- o Pencil and sketchbook
- o Music sheet and instrument
- o Welding tools and metal
- o Melodic beats and a dance routine
- o Yarn and knitting needles
- o Paint palette and easel
- o Garden trowel and fresh dirt
- o Laptop and coding sequences
- o Piece of wood and saw or router
- o Material and needle with thread
- o Nature and time with your camera

During the creative process (whatever that looks like for you) your brain releases dopamine - a natural antidepressant. You tend to experience higher self-esteem and sense of accomplishment as you create something meaningful to you.

"To be creative is to let little pieces of your heart go,
and place them into each project you make."
~ Pat Bravo ~

Have you ever noticed that if you're fully engaged in a creative process, you feel more at peace? You're less focused on external stimuli or the dozen thoughts swirling around your head, and more centered on personal thoughts and feelings. Creativity can be a driving force in opening up to self-reflection.

The most important thing you need to do here is get past any limiting belief that screams out "you're not creative!" It's a belief that I held onto for a long time myself. I equated creativity to being able to create a watercolour masterpiece - a skill that I may be able to learn, but it most definitely does not come naturally. If you look at the list I shared, I bet you can identify with at least one activity, or maybe you already have your own creative outlet.

I've chosen to dig a little deeper into the world of journaling with pen and paper in this chapter. Although other modes of creativity can achieve the same results, there is something undeniably important about healing through expressing words. The only challenge you'll face is a limiting belief such as:

"I don't write. Keeping journals just doesn't work for me."

I hear this statement so often that I debated about removing journaling from the Healing Compass. But writing and the power of words have had such a profound effect on me and my journey that I had to include it. Everyone should give it a shot at the very least.

Sometimes the challenge may be that we don't know what to write, or we don't have a starting point. Or we may hold ourselves back by worrying that the words we put on paper might be shared with the rest of the world one day.

Realize that your words are for you. And you alone. Put a clause in your will that states your journals are to be buried with you. And threaten to haunt anyone who goes against that wish. You can also get rid of your words after you write them down. There's no rule that says you have to hold on to everything that you write. You make the rules.

"It's like whispering to one's self and listening at the same time."
~ Mina Murray ~

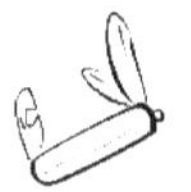 *Your Tools:*

→ **Write It In A Letter**

This is the easiest way for me to get going. I like it because it's conversational and the words flow out of me easier than if I sit down and try to work through and unpack a particular emotion or experience.

Here are some examples:

> (A letter to my younger self - after a time of feeling sad for the teenage girl who felt so alone)
>
> *Dear Angie,*
>
> *I wish I could go back and hold your hand through all of those difficult high school years. I wish that I could tell you that even though you're lonely and want so badly to just fit in, you're learning to navigate through this loneliness in a beautiful way and in a few years you're going to find your people. Your tribe. You'll connect with familiar people and new people in ways that you wouldn't be able to if you were that "popular" person that you desperately wish to be right now.*

> (A letter to my present self - after feeling fear about jumping so far outside of my comfort zone)
>
> *Dear Angie,*
>
> *You're rocking life right now. Don't forget that. The days get so busy and fly by - maybe stop for a moment to reflect on that shy, awkward little girl you once were. Honour her and remember that she is still a part of you, no matter how far you've come. Think about the confident, happy woman that you've grown into and honour her. Be kind to her. There are days where she feels like a really crappy mom or a bad friend. Hold her hand and look into her eyes to tell her that she's amazing and doing the best with everything.*

See? Your words don't have to be profound. Grammar doesn't matter. Honesty does.

It turns out that writing letters to myself has been more healing than I ever would have imagined. You see, I listen really well to myself when the words are on paper. I read and re-read them, stopping to reflect. It's one of the rare times where self-compassion comes so easy.

→ **Gratitude Journals**

Have you ever kept a Gratitude Journal? Taking a few minutes out of your day to write down what you're grateful for? This simple exercise, often so simple that people skip right over it, is the most powerful journaling technique that I've ever found.

First thing in the morning, write down three things you're grateful for. That's it. Same as before, this doesn't have to be profound. I wake up some days, feeling sick and exhausted, and the only three things I can think of are:

- o   I can still breathe
- o   We have lots of coffee[16]
- o   Our house is warm

Like I said, not profound. Other days I can dig a little deeper, but the truth is that it doesn't matter - giving thanks for something, every single day, is a simple journaling act that will bring an abundance of positive energy into your life.

→ **One Line a Day**

Journaling doesn't even have to dig down deep into feelings and emotions. It can be a simple sentence that describes something you did or felt today. Start it in a journal (even a simple notebook that has enough pages for the whole year). At the top of each page write the day (January 1 for example), and then on the first line write the current year (2018 for example). After that headline, write down your one sentence memory, or feeling. Work your way through the whole year, and then next year start with a new headline (2019) with your new memory or feeling.

The brilliance behind this journaling technique is that it leads

---

[16] Priorities, right?

into reflection and positive emotions when you remember the things you experienced in the years past. And it only takes 30 seconds out of your day. Period.

"Start writing, no matter what.
The water doesn't flow until the faucet is turned on."
~ Louis L'Amour ~

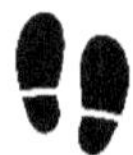 ## Your Next Steps:

→ **Start with gratitude.** It really is empowering. In a notebook, a dusty journal that's been sitting on your shelf, or on post-it notes - write down three things every morning that you're grateful for. This will have an amazing effect on your emotional health, even on the days where it feels repetitive and mundane.

"Don't forget - no one else sees the world the way you do, so no one else can tell the stories that you have to tell."
~ Charles de Lint ~

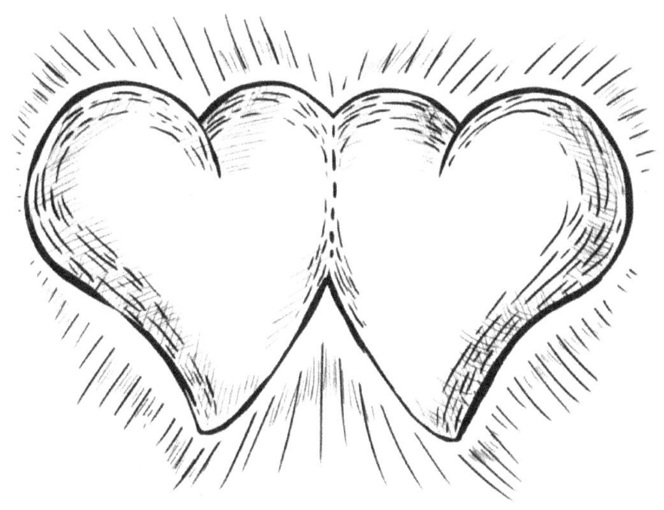

Connect the Dots

"Love your family. Spend time, be kind, and serve one another. Tomorrow isn't promised and today is short."
~ Unknown ~

Our living room is alive with three different conversations. Some cousins catch up on the months that have passed by since they last chatted, a grandma listens to the excited antics of her grandson, and two couples who have just met for the first time share stories of their travels.

Meanwhile, the kitchen smells like freshly baked pizza as my dear cousin helps me assemble the last pizza concoctions. My husband stops by with two glasses of wine and helps me slice and serve the first couple of pizzas, while we continue to rotate more of them in and out of the oven.

Half a dozen kids run through the kitchen giggling, en route to the toys downstairs and the doorbell rings with some more guests arriving. I love that we rarely have to answer the door. Our friends and family feel welcome enough to come on in, simply using the doorbell as an announcement that they've arrived.

This is one of our pizza parties. We have them regularly, on the first Friday of the month, skipping a couple of months where people are generally too busy. The tradition was born out of a place of disconnection, a time in my life where my chronic illness made socializing with family and friends difficult and our kids were so little that schlepping them around everywhere was not our idea of fun.

We desperately wanted to see our friends and family more and since I love hosting and planning parties, our Pizza Party tradition came alive. Every month we send an invite out to friends and family, knowing that everyone has busy schedules and people will make it when they can. It's wonderful, as we have a completely different turnout and combination of people each and every month. We make the pizzas ourselves, and I've become skilled at sourcing the ingredients to keep costs low. It may sound like a lot of work, but it really isn't. It's been the easiest and most enjoyable way to connect with so many of our friends and family.

Connecting with loved ones is one of the simplest things we can do to help our Hearts heal, yet like so many other things, it's sometimes easier said than done.

It's one of life's great mysteries that during times of stress and overwhelm, right when we need connection the most, we tend to become even more disconnected. When emotions and pain start to overrule our lives, our instinct is often to push connection away, even though our hearts are screaming for someone to hold our hand and kiss our wounds.

Why? Isn't that the most backward way to act? Why do we push away this support and love? There are many reasons. But quite simply, isn't it easier to tell someone that you're doing "just fine" than to expose a piece of your heart?

We wear masks and build brick walls to protect our hearts, because being vulnerable is scary and unknown territory. Social media has made this worse by replacing real life, face-to-face interaction. We need to counteract this trend by committing to spend more time with each other around a kitchen table, and less time behind a screen.

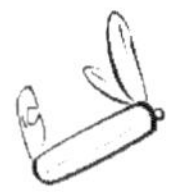 ## Your Tools:

→ **Love and Honor Your Rocks:** Your inner circle. The relationships that blossom when you're being authentic and genuine. The people that are there for you in the worst of times. Take time for those relationships. Give your time to those friends and family members and receive their time and listening ears in return. Give-give relationships are the only kind that will flourish.

→ **Make Rituals**: I love this part. Start planning things in your calendar that run on clockwork so that you can nurture some of your relationships on a more regular basis.

   o **Friend Getaways:** My best friend and I have a Mommy Getaway every year where we take time out of our busy schedules to have a night away in the mountains. We rent a condo, bring food to munch on, wine to share, and talk for hours and hours on end. We both receive extensive emotional healing from this time together.

   o **Date Night:** Connecting with your other half has to be a priority, despite how busy and crazy life can get. My husband and I take our monthly couples massage dates seriously and prioritize them above most other things. We treat ourselves to dinner afterwards, and the uninterrupted conversations we have allow us to feel both seen and heard in our relationship.

   o **Kids One on One:** We do a lot with our kids but focusing on the one-on-one part of the equation has been a game-changer. As we go on coffee/hot chocolate dates with our oldest daughter, build Lego with our son, or play tea party with our youngest, we often chat about school, friends, their worries, and their dreams. It fills all of our hearts with more compassion and understanding.

→ **Find Your Army:** Whatever you may be struggling with in life, it's important to find people who have been on a similar path. You need the strength and support you get from your Rocks, but you need the empathy and compassion that you get from your Army as well. My Army includes some members of my local ostomy support group, including the two ladies that came to see me in the hospital when I had my first surgery. Lisa & Sheri were instrumental to my emotional healing on that leg of my journey, and they've become lifelong friends. Through that same support group, I found Paula and Kaylee. We have just as many differences between us as similarities, yet our bond is undeniably strong. When someone understands because they have literally walked a mile in your shoes[17], that compassion is a deep source of healing.

Finding your Army doesn't just relate to illness or disease. What about your passions? Are you a photographer? Have you ever tried meeting up with a group of fellow photographers and found an instant bond and friendship as you discuss your worst client experiences and share tips and tricks of the trade? Or maybe you're a runner? Have you ever joined a running club and found just as much pleasure in the post-run snacks and drinks you meet up for, as you do with the run itself? Talking to somebody else who just "gets it" makes a world of difference.

"I define connection as the energy that exists between people when they feel seen, heard, and valued; when they can give and receive without judgment; and when they derive sustenance and strength from the relationship."
~ Brené Brown ~

When I think of myself as the central point in a diagram, connecting the dots to all of the important relationships I have in my life, I smile at the eclectic group of characters it includes. That's the best part - I have found my collection of close friends and family members that are living their true, authentic lives. This makes all of them different and unique, which creates the most beautiful picture in my mind of my tribe.

---

[17] Or 7,000, as the case may be...

 **Inspired By...**

Brené Brown: This amazing lady has been a mentor of mine for a long time. I devour every book she writes and gain incredible insight and wisdom in the process. (*The Gifts of Imperfection, Daring Greatly, Rising Strong,* and *Braving the Wilderness*). One of the simplest ways to see some of the work she's done is to watch one of her talks on YouTube. Her 2011 TED Talk, "The Power of Vulnerability", has been viewed over 7 million times. It's powerful, as is all of her work. You could also watch a short, three minute video called "Brené Brown on Blame" - it will make you laugh and nod your head in complete understanding, as we have all walked a mile in those shoes.

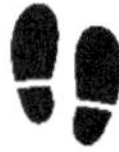 *Your Next Steps:*

→ **Banish the words "oh, fine" and "pretty good" from your vocabulary.** Practice being genuine and authentic with your feelings and what's going on in your life.

→ **Make a list of the relationships closest to you.** Beside each person jot down something that you could do to reach out to them. **Keep it simple.** Send a card in the mail, give them a call, put that coffee date into the calendar, or plan a dinner. Think about rituals you can build to help nurture these connections.

"Find your tribe. Love them hard."
~ *Unknown* ~

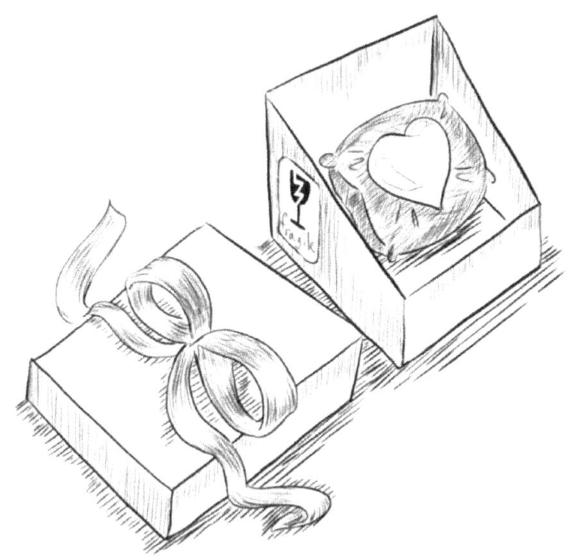

A New Kind of Self-Care

"Perhaps, we should love ourselves so fiercely,
that when others see us they know
exactly how it should be done."
~ Rudy Francisco ~

Self-care is important. You won't hear me debate that fact. I'm kind of new to the game, and in many ways I am very much a rookie. What I can say though, is that as I try to become better-versed and more experienced with the practice of self-care, I start to worry about all of the fakers out there, including myself.

I faked it for years. This is the self-care I used to practice:
- o Self-care = having a bubble bath
- o Self-care = taking "me time" to watch a TV show
- o Self-care = buying myself a fancy, yummy coffee

What makes it fake self-care? If the act itself doesn't provide real rest and rejuvenation, or if the act itself doesn't promote self-compassion and self-acceptance - then it's not self-care.

Let's dig a little deeper...
- o Was the 60 minute bubble bath relaxing? Yeah, kind of. But did I gain an ounce of self-compassion while I continued to build my to-do list in my head and over-analyze my interactions with my kids that day? No.
- o Was the TV show rejuvenating? Not really, as I zoned out with two glasses of wine, avoiding some uncomfortable feelings I should work through.
- o How about that yummy latte? My Instagram picture might show a beautiful cup of coffee with the hashtag #selfcaresaturday. Yet it doesn't show my frustration with the long lineup or the overwhelm I felt with so much noise inside the coffee shop.

I've recently changed my view and value of self-care. Today, I believe that to understand it better, I have to dig a little (or a lot) deeper. Self-care doesn't belong on the surface. We can't just dabble in it on a superficial level. We have to get down into the trenches, exploring self-compassion and self-acceptance.

Now, I call this self-love. That's the art I practice, and it truly is an art - the more you practice it, the better you get at it.

"You owe yourself the love that you so freely give to other people."
~ Unknown ~

I didn't discover how much I sucked at practicing self-care until a memorable visit with my therapist one Tuesday evening. She asked me the exact same question she'd been asking for three weeks and I responded in the exact same way.

Therapist: "So, how did things go this week with finding a pocket of time for yourself?"
Me: "It was a crazy week. Life has been so busy lately. I will definitely plan to do something this week."
Therapist: *(nodding in that quiet way that they must teach in therapist school)* "Why do you think that everyone else is more important than you are? Where does that come from?"
Me: "Oh, I'm important. I just need to find more time, things will slow down soon." *(I half questioned, half promised her)*
[pregnant pause]
Therapist: "What would you think about your daughter being in this same chair in 15 years, telling me that she doesn't have the time in her schedule to take care of herself?"

Well…. that stung. Tears sprung to my eyes, and as I half sobbed my response, I told her in no uncertain terms that would never happen. Because I would make sure that it didn't. And as the words blubbered out of my mouth, even I didn't believe a single word that I said.

Turns out that was the exact kick in the pants I needed. I woke up the next day, believing for the first time ever that in order to be the best mom and wife that I could be, I would first have to become the best Me that I could be. To do that, my Heart and Soul needed a little tending to.

I searched for a pocket of time that I could use to do the things that would fill my heart with self-love. What worked best was early in the morning, before the rest of the house was up. It felt a little crazy at first, getting up between 5:00 and 6:00 in the morning to practice self-care through various activities. But it didn't take long before I was hooked.

I discovered the things that connected with me through

reading some books on the topic (I share those in the "Inspired By" section), and exploring the idea of finding an activity to help heal each area of the Healing Compass.

"Your entire life changes the day that you decide you will no longer accept mediocrity for yourself. When you realize that today is the most important day of your life."
~ Hal Elrod ~

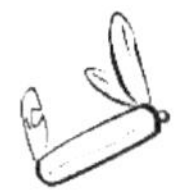 *Your Tools:*

→ **Food for the Soul:** I start off the day with meditating. Or I spend a couple of minutes taking deep breaths, letting the air reach deep into my belly.

→ **Food for the Heart:** I write down three things I'm grateful for. Then as a bonus boost for my heart, I read a simple affirmation to myself 5-10 times. I usually read it out loud, in a quiet whisper to make the words have more of an impact. The sentence is simple, and I have a list of favourites that I cycle through. Some examples:
  → "I am enough."
  → "There is a stream of love supporting my dreams."
  → "I believe in the person I am becoming."
If you're new to the world of affirmations and think they're "woo-woo-hippie-stuff"[18], just give them a shot. You might be surprised at how much self-love you start feeling after trying them for a few weeks.

→ **Food for the Mind:** I turn to the latest personal development book that I'm reading and try to finish at least one chapter,

---

[18] My exact definition before I started using them

but if I only have 5 minutes and can get through a handful of pages, then that's okay too.

→ **Food for the Body:** A little bit of movement starts me off on the right foot. I tend to save a bigger chunk of exercise for later on in the day, but in my morning routine I'll do some simple stretches or a short yoga routine (sun salutations are my fave).

I can complete these steps in anywhere from 15-30 minutes, depending on how much time I have in my early morning. The impact these self-care steps have on the rest of my day is huge.

"Rest and self-care are so important. When you take time to replenish your spirit, it allows you to serve others from the overflow. You cannot serve from an empty vessel."
~ *Eleanor Brownn* ~

Reflecting back to when I began focusing on my physical health, my main motivation was the realization that I was the sole person responsible for taking care of the only Body I have. Similarly, sitting in my therapist's office that day I realized that there was nobody else who was going to take care of my stressed out, too-busy, hustle-bustle Heart. This woke me up fast and hard.

I used to "kind-of" like myself. I gave my Heart the same amount of attention as I would give the charming, yet annoying salesman that comes to the door. Too polite to turn him away, but too annoyed to give him my time or energy. Now, with some work and a change in perspective, I am truly, head-over-heels in love with myself. I still get annoyed with some quirks here and there, like we always will, but I love Me and will always find the time to take care of this Heart of mine.

 **Inspired By...**

Shauna Niequist: As I read her book *Present Over Perfect*, I silently sobbed, nodding my head the entire time, feeling like somebody had insight into the inner workings of my soul. Shauna digs deep into the ideas of self-compassion and self-love as she describes her journey from a frantic, over-packed life to one filled with more grace, silence, and simplicity.

Hal Elrod: His book, *The Miracle Morning*, introduced me to the idea of carving out time in my day before anyone else was up to take care of myself. The routine I follow is based on the S.A.V.E.R.S. routine he outlines in detail in his book and on his website. According to the thousands of people who have offered a review of his book - this same routine has changed the lives of many people around the world.

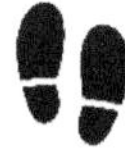 *Your Next Steps:*

→ Set your alarm to wake up 30 minutes early, and use that early morning time to practice one or two self-love tools.

"Choose every day, to forgive yourself.
You are human, flawed, and most of all worthy of love."
~ Alison Malee ~

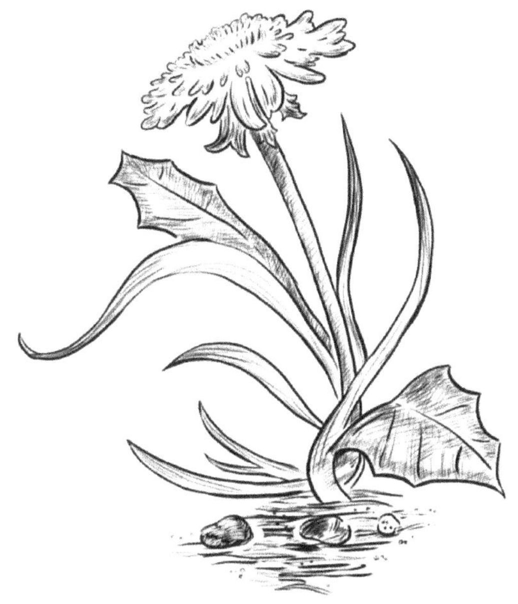

Finding Dandelions

"The greatest weapon against stress is our ability to choose one thought over another."
~ *William James* ~

"You have the best outlook on life," friends and family tell me, referring to my optimistic candor and choice to see the bright side of the challenges and struggles I've faced. That's the side of me that I choose to put on social media and share in the time spent with the people in my life.

It doesn't mean that it comes naturally. You see, that's the side of me that I **choose** to show the rest of the world. What they don't see is the behind the scenes stuff that leads up to that cheerful, positive presentation of myself. It's not fake. I really am optimistic and want to find joy and light where I can, but it's important that everyone realizes that we all have this choice in life.

I've been in the depths of loss and grief. I've been in the valley of being so ill that the prospect of dying didn't seem like such a bad deal. That's not tongue in cheek. It's a truth that I haven't admitted to very many people. And it's a reality for most people living lives with chronic pain and chronic fatigue, or lives consumed by anxiety or depression.

It took intentional steps to get to the other side of those dark times in my life. Understanding that joy or sadness was my choice every day when I woke up, gave me the push to always want to choose joy. To choose light. And to choose love.

"Dave's death changed me in very profound ways. I learned about the depths of sadness and the brutality of loss. But I also learned that when life sucks you under, you can kick against the bottom, break the surface, and breathe again. I learned that in the face of the void - or in the face of any challenge - you can choose joy and meaning."
~ Sheryl Sandberg ~

This chapter is called Finding Dandelions because of a legacy my dad left behind. My decision to move my life forward by choosing joy every single day, came from the heartache and grief of losing one of the most important people in my life.

When my dad was first diagnosed with cancer, I had to receive the devastating news from my home two hours away. My mom had called my husband first to share the news with him and asked him to be with me when I found out. So he held me as he shared the heartache that had been handed to my parents and siblings earlier that day. After sobbing into his arms for a while, I reached for the phone to call my mom and dad. Mom talked to me first and then handed the phone to Dad. He was somber but had that upbeat tone to his voice that he always had. "It is what it is. We'll fight until we can't anymore," he told me.

I was almost seven months pregnant at the time and we were also only six months into fostering our 5 year old little girl who we would later adopt. Life was busy and challenging as we navigated the next few months by spending every moment we could with my dad, while still working through the realities of life you can't put on hold - childbirth, an autoimmune flare-up, life with a newborn, and learning how to nurture and help our little girl. Dad passed away less than five months after that diagnosis. And he was a man of his word, he fought until he couldn't anymore.

There was a smile on his face and shining from his soul, even in his last 24 hours before cancer made that smile only a memory.

I used to think of my dad as the eternal optimist. He would see the good in every situation. On Winter Solstice, the shortest day of the year when everyone is complaining about how little daylight there is and how the cold winter lays ahead of us, my dad would always say "it just gets better from here," referring to every day getting longer and bringing us closer to warmer temps and summer in a few months time.

Every time there was something that I felt like complaining a little about - a university midterm, the latest bout of the flu, or just some crappy weather - my dad would say "it could always be worse." Never in a condescending way - he always listened to my worries and concerns, but then offered a friendly reminder that we always have something to be grateful for.

He would point out our dining room window to a field covered with yellow dandelions and say, "have you seen my rose garden?" He always referred to the dandelions as his yellow roses, and he made it his mission every spring to find the first ones in our yard. He'd pick them and bring them into my mom - his yellow roses. She'd roll her eyes with a loving grin on her face and tell him she'd appreciate real roses one day.

These yellow roses have become a family legacy. My dad's optimism lives on in every family member as we continue to work through struggles, challenges and tough times in all of our lives.

Working my way through grieving the loss of my dad, and then having that loss tear an even larger hole when cancer took my sister's life, has forced me to struggle with optimism at times.

I have wanted so badly to follow in my dad's footsteps and share all of the optimism he had with the rest of the world. His outlook on life is something the entire world needs more of - but something was missing. It was so hard to share this optimism when I struggled to deal with the devastation, anger, and hurt that I felt inside.

And then I realized that my dad didn't just see the good in everything - he chose to acknowledge the bad, recognize the hurt, see the "weeds" in life instead of just moving past them. Then, he would choose joy. He would push past the struggles and the tough times, and choose to live life with happiness in his heart.

Finding Dandelions has become a metaphor in my life that has woven itself into every single one of my days. We can choose to walk by and push past all of these annoying, ugly things in our life - the weeds. Or we can see them and appreciate the fact that we can still find gratitude amongst the weeds.

"Every experience, no matter how bad it seems, holds within it a blessing of some kind. The goal is to find it."
~ Buddha ~

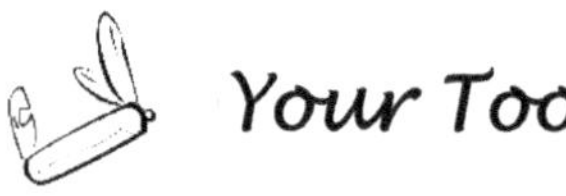 **Your Tools:**

→ **Look for Dandelions:** These are the things in our lives that might normally cause frustration or disappointment, or ignite sadness or anger. Identify those things that weigh on your heart, that cause more negative emotions than positive ones. Sit with the negative emotion for a short while. Sadness, anger, frustration, and disappointment are all healthy emotions to feel when we have the intention of moving through them towards love and joy.

→ **Choose Joy:** Now, try to look for what makes the dandelion beautiful. I look for weeds, and try to see them as flowers. This will have a profound effect on your ability to process all sorts of emotions.

→ **Remember That You Are in Control:** You hold the power of choosing how you feel, how you react, and what emotions you hold on to or let free. It takes effort and it takes practice, but realizing that you are the master of your outlook on life is a liberating feeling.

"Life is ironic. It takes sadness to know what happiness is, noise to appreciate silence, and absence to value presence."
~ Unknown ~

The important part to remember is that we should acknowledge the hurt and see the pain. We can't just brush it under a rug, or worse yet store it in a bottle on our overflowing "emotion" shelves. We have to be okay with having a bad day once in a while. The key words being "once in a while". Then we need to realize that it is completely **our choice** how we continue on. We can choose joy, we can choose love, and we can find the dandelions.

❤ Inspired By...

> **Mom & Dad:** My favourite mentors, teachers and source of inspiration. My ability to work through every challenging thing in my life comes from what I have learned from them. They didn't teach by sitting me down and telling me about the importance of choosing to see the good in life amongst the weeds. However they did teach by example, and they have both set an amazing one.

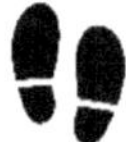 Your Next Steps:

→ Make it your mission to find a dandelion every day for a month. That's 30 negative experiences or feelings that you can start to see the positive in.

→ Allow a bad day to happen. You don't want too many of these, but the next time you feel sad, let yourself feel sad in a way that works for you. And then remind yourself that you are the only person who has control of your thoughts. Take that sense of control and choose joy.

"The sun is a daily reminder that we too can rise again from the darkness, that we too can shine our own light."
~ S. Ajna ~

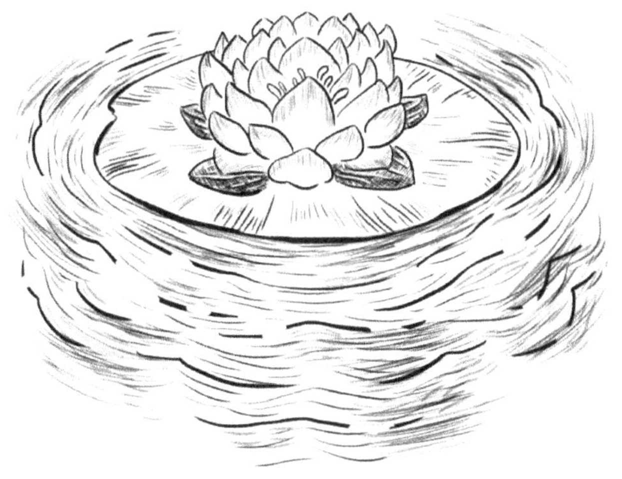

Your Soul

(Section Four)

"Accept what is, let go of what was,
and believe in what will be."
~ Unknown ~

If it were up to me, my Soul is the area I would focus my energy on all day, every day. But darn it, those kids need to be fed and life just keeps getting in the way. However, it's become so important to me that I make it my priority first thing every morning. But on the days when I'm not able to fit in time for tending to my soul, I find that I'm more sluggish, more easily irritated, and quite honestly not the best mom and wife that I can be.

What is spiritual health? At a basic level it's your inner connection with yourself. It's knowing yourself at a deeper, more intimate level, and loving the person you are deep down.

I'll be honest with you - I don't always love my surface-level self, especially the version of me that shows up when my health and happiness are totally out of balance. She's a little "crazy" - that Angie. However, I am totally in love with my deep-down self. Finding her wasn't necessarily easy, but very much worth it.

"you have to find that place
that brings out the human in you.
the soul in you. the love in you."
~ r.m. drake ~

Spiritual health is knowing that you have a purpose, and you are willing to work on your passions and skills to leave your mark on the world, be it large or small. Sometimes people get too caught up in the idea that changing the world for the better means solving big issues like world hunger. Nope. Be a good person, help others, and spread love not hate. There is no doubt that you will influence at least one person, or maybe ten, or maybe even a hundred. Then, as those people move through their lives with the same mission - trying to change the world for the better - amazing ripple effects happen.

When you become spiritually healthy, you:
- o   Feel harmony in your life
- o   Feel compassion towards others and engage in altruistic

acts
- o Can articulate your values and life goals
- o Work towards those goals, giving your life purpose and direction
- o Know how to sit in silence comfortably

"Get the inside right. The outside will fall into place."
~ Eckhart Tolle ~

We live in a chaotic world. We're surrounded by outer noise and we tend to internalize a ton of inner noise. Our souls need more quiet.

At the very center of it all, you need to fall in love with the life you're living. And to do that you need to be creating the life you want to have. Spiritual healing comes from the values, dreams, and goals you have inside of you. And you are the only one that can bring those values to life, make your dreams come true, and achieve every goal you set for yourself.

What are you going to work on in this section?

Can You Hear That? You need to become familiar and comfortable with silence. Meditation is an excellent tool.
Be Here Now: You must love Today, not fret about Yesterday or worry about Tomorrow.
Get In The Driver's Seat: You are 100% in charge of creating the life of your dreams.
Grow Your Give Muscle: Learn that giving is so much more healing than receiving and decide where you want to give back to the world.
Back to Nature: Spend time with the trees and see the stars in person - that's enough to bring huge amounts of healing into your Soul.

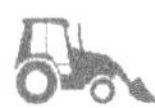

Bring Out the Backhoe...

Travel... (without the computer in your pocket)
This is a two part process and both parts are equally important. The first step is to travel. And this doesn't have to equal jumping on an airplane and exploring somewhere foreign, on the other side of the globe. You can travel an hour away from home and discover a place that you've never seen before. It helps if it can be one step outside of your comfort zone – think along the lines of a hike you've never done before or visiting a city whose transit system you're unfamiliar with.

Step two is to slow down and explore this new place without the distraction of that tiny computer we all carry around with us. Turn your phone off and keep it for emergency purposes only. Now, open your eyes and see things for the first time. Use your five senses to touch, see, smell, taste, and listen to everything around you. If you are in a city, find your way around by asking strangers for directions. Try a new food and strike up conversation with the waiter or waitress asking them about their town or city. If you're out in the wilderness, really slow down. Don't focus on the kilometres left to travel or the to-do list that won't stop popping into your mind. Take a deep breath of that fresh, crisp air and spend time with your thoughts, really taking time to listen to what your Soul is whispering to you when the noise is gone.

These two experiences might sound contradictory to each other – one in the hustle-bustle of a city, and the other in the quiet of the great outdoors. But they're both instrumental to healing your Soul. They both connect you to the greater world around you, and help you feel refreshed and renewed. With that deeper connection to the world **around** you, you will start feeling a deeper connection to the world **within** you as well.

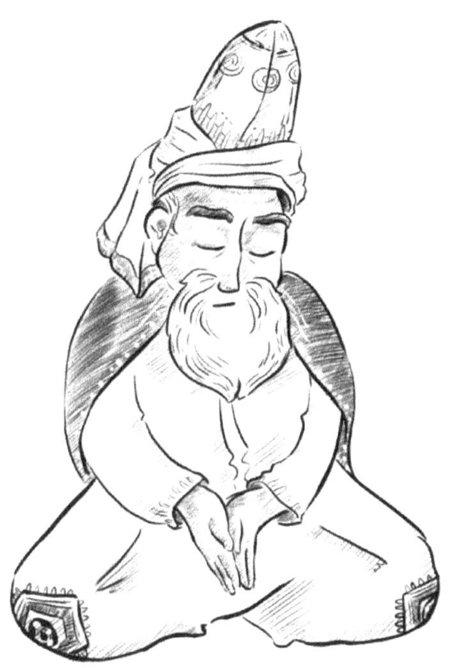

Can You Hear That?

"Listen to silence.
It has so much to say."
~ Rumi ~

I used to suck at meditating. And since honesty and vulnerability are key here, let me admit - I fake meditated for years.

Oh my gosh, that looks even more lame written down than it sounded in my head, but it's true.

During those first few years of handling illness, I knew that the act of meditation would be beneficial for my health. I was completing my second university degree, working part-time, and trying my hardest to be as "normal" as possible despite my body breaking down all around me. I had high hopes that meditation would help ground and centre me.

So at first I did what all good bookworms would do, I found half a dozen meditation books and an audio CD of guided meditations at my local library. I was going to master this, easy peasy. There's a strong likelihood that one of those books was Meditation for Dummies. That's how beginner I was.

I tried following the advice. I listened to a guide walk me step by step through what I should be doing. I focused on my breathing. Ten minutes felt like *forever...* I pictured a happy place, usually sitting on some rocks by a rushing river. And every time my mind wandered, I tried to refocus on my breath and to just "let those thoughts go with ease."

This was my hiccup. Let them "go with ease"? What does that even mean? My monkey mind could not handle it. The thoughts wouldn't stop. Ever. They just kept coming - everything from "I think we're running low on milk" to "what am I doing with my life?". I felt like I ended my meditation sessions with more frustration about my innate inability to "just be", than with peace in my soul.

Eventually Fate decided to give me some help.[19] I found Headspace.

Headspace is an app that teaches meditation and mindfulness in the most impressive, down-to-the basics way possible. Andy Puddicombe is the meditation master whose voice you hear throughout the various programs, and I'm pretty sure he's right inside my head as he gently guides me back to a place of quiet

---

[19] Or was it Google Ads? Hard to say...

and calm whenever my mind wanders.

I've learned that I don't need to completely stop the mental chatter, but I can note when it's there and then return focus to my breathing. My meditation journey has reached far beyond just wanting to find a quiet space in my mind, as I've worked my way through different series on Productivity, Stress, Relationships, and Motivation. There are many other options as well. Taking ten minutes in the morning to meditate has become one of my favourite parts of the day.

"Meditation is not a way of making your mind quiet.
It's a way of entering into the quiet that's already there."
~ Deepak Chopra ~

Learning how to meditate, and making it a regular habit, has had a profound effect on my health and happiness. The largest change is helping me with emotional regulation.

The old Me needed a version of nuclear reactor warning labels to warn friends and family of my tendency to react strongly and disproportionately to many different scenarios, no matter how small. For example, my husband suggesting a change in plans to our weekend could result in tears welling up in my eyes and my voice cracking as I tried to explain why I felt our original plan worked better.

The sole reason for those tears and crackly voice were my inability to recognize just what emotion I was feeling. It would bubble up over the surface before I even knew I had a feeling about the particular subject. My over-reactions were not only frustrating for my loved ones, but they drove me crazy as well. "I don't know why I'm crying..." became something I said almost daily.

I dealt with situations like this multiple times a day, and usually only with those closest to me. The closer you were, the more you saw the over-emotional reactions to the smallest of things. All because I had no skills in regulating my emotions, or being able to identify them.

After meditating regularly, I started recognizing those emotions as they bubbled up and would stop to take a moment to breathe. Simply asking myself "what's going on here?" and taking a pause gave me the power to respond appropriately rather than react as soon as I felt an emotion.

Learning emotional regulation has saved our marriage, as living with a nuclear reactor wife isn't very fun. I'm also much better equipped to help our kids with these skills.

"I do not fix my problems. I fix my thinking.
Then problems fix themselves."
~ Louise Hay ~

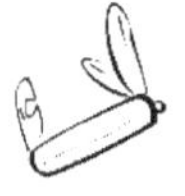 ## Your Tools:

Here are my top three suggestions for meditation guides based on what has worked best for me:

→ **Headspace:** You can get started for free with their 10 day introduction to the program through their app on your phone. If you like it, you can subscribe for a monthly or annual fee, or you could also continue using those 10 free lessons over and over again. I originally balked at the cost, but when it worked out to the cost of a couple of coffees per month, I realized that I would never question paying that for a gym membership, and then my perspective shifted.

→ **Calm App:** This is rated as the #1 app for mindfulness and meditation. It combines meditations with breathing exercises and relaxing music to fall asleep to. It also has a free introduction side to it, or you can subscribe annually for a minimal monthly cost.

→ **Self-Care for Busy People:** This is a meditation album created by Kris Carr of the *Crazy Sexy* series of books. I have the tracks saved on my phone and it's my go-to when I feel myself heading down the self-doubt or self-sabotage road. Personally, I love that she calls me sweetie and encourages me with beautiful affirmations full of self-love.

"Where there is peace and meditation,
there is neither anxiety nor doubt."
~ St. Francis de Sales ~

Learning how to sit in silence, focusing on my breathing rather than on the million thoughts in my head, was a big discovery on my roadmap to better health. I have no doubt that it would make a difference in the lives of every single person on the planet. It has reduced stress in my life, helped me with anxiety, given me tools for relationships, and increased my concentration and focus. When I reflect on the high value of those benefits, I have no problem justifying the cost of paying for a meditation guide.

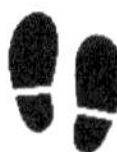 Your Next Steps:

→ Try it. It's that simple. Don't run out and buy something if it doesn't work for you, but try the free side of the tools I suggested or find one that works for you.

"I think 99 times and I find nothing. I stop thinking,
swim in silence, and the truth comes to me."
~ Albert Einstein ~

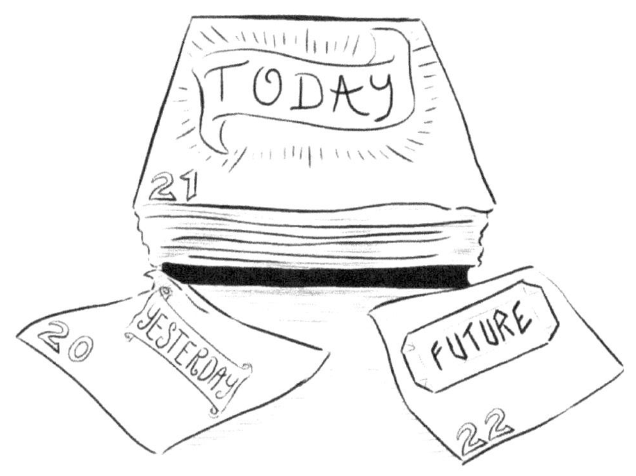

Be Here Now

"There are only two days in the year that nothing can be done. One is called yesterday and the other is called tomorrow. So today is the right day to love, believe, do and mostly live."
~ Dalai Lama ~

Three words flash before my eyes as I pick up my phone randomly throughout the day. A carefully selected screen saver with vibrant colours in the background and these bold words on top: Be Here Now.

9 times out of 10, I set my phone back down again because I don't need to be checking email or scrolling through social media at that very moment. Usually what I need is a connection in the real world. Not the cyber world.

I chose that screensaver on my phone so that I could be much more intentional about my life. When I'm with my kids, I can focus on really being *with* them. When I'm tackling housework, I stop getting distracted by the 11 things running around my monkey mind. And the hardest one to master - when I'm having Me Time, I need to stop doing other things and really focus on doing something restful and rejuvenating for myself.

Those three simple words have become my motto, and each word has become symbolic on its own in my day-to-day life. I need to just **be**, carefully setting down the seven balls I'm juggling and focus on one at a time. I have to appreciate **here**, eliminating comparison and loving the life I have. And I need to believe that **now** is the only time I have, embracing and loving today, each and every day.

"Worrying does not take away tomorrow's troubles.
It takes away today's peace."
~ *Randy Armstrong* ~

Life is too short. The older I get and the more loss I experience, the greater this truth becomes a reality. Having this reality build deeper roots into my life has really helped me become intentional about living in the present moment, not the past or future. The past can sometimes haunt us, stealing our time away as we fret and over-analyze various situations and memories. Likewise, the future can be just as greedy, carving hours out of our days with worry and anxiety about things that haven't even happened yet.

This practice of living in the present moment is called mindfulness. The more I thought about it, the more I realized how important it was for me to start practicing this skill.

One of my biggest challenges unveiled itself right away. I believe it's a challenge that most of us face. I was trying to multi-task every single area of my life. I used to think of multi-tasking as the glorious answer to bring productivity and purpose to every part of my life. And for a while I fooled myself into believing that I could manage like that. Probably because I truly believed that everyone else was excelling at it.

After all, it should make perfect sense to be the best wife, mom, employee, friend, homemaker, volunteer, and person, with the skills needed to juggle those seven balls in the air, all while honing the perfect body, the most intelligent mind, and a giving heart. Oh, and walking the dog. Let's not forget that.

The need to be all the things and do all the things is a problem that plagues so many people.

The truth is multi-tasking is a farce. Except for the most mundane of tasks - I can fold laundry and listen to a podcast at the same time. However, I can't "mom" and "wife" at the same time. It's impossible to give my husband the attention he deserves as he's sharing a new work challenge, while we're interrupted by the kids 37 times with every question and near-disaster under the sun.

So now I one-task. You may want to call it uni-task but that makes me think of a unitard, and that drives me crazy. This fits in perfectly with the blocks of time I created in the chapter Boss of the Clock. When I have my Kid Block, and my only role to focus on is being their mom, I can spend my time and energy being a much better one. When I'm in a Friend Block and trying to have a conversation on the phone with a dear friend that I haven't chatted with in six months, I'm likely plunking my kids in front of the TV and randomly tossing snacks their way every time they try to interrupt me. Perhaps not my best mom moment, but that's ok because I make sure that I am a great mom when it matters.

To make the best use of one-tasking and learning to live in the present moment, I've had to learn two particular tools and practice them regularly. I accept life as it is, and I let go of everything not useful for me.

"There are things that we don't want to happen but have to accept,
things we don't want to know but have to learn,
and people we can't live without but have to let go."
~ Unknown ~

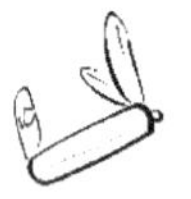 **Your Tools:**

→ **Acceptance:** Practice this phrase, "It is, as it is". And I have another secret for you, accepting things "as is" doesn't mean you have to like things as they are. Don't attach a feeling to acceptance if you don't want to.

Let's imagine an example. You receive a pay-cut at work because the economy is struggling. It sucks. There's no way to get around the fact that this change may cause hard times in your life, an adjustment of priorities, and cutting some expenses out of your day-to-day budget. Accepting that this "is as it is" doesn't mean brushing your hurt and disappointment under a rug and re-framing it as a blessing. You can feel that hurt and that disappointment. You need to feel those things. Remember the cautionary Emotional Bottling tale? But you don't need to attach worry, and stay up all night creating imaginary scenarios of devastation that haven't happened yet.

Accepting any situation "as is" means telling yourself that you can't solve the problem in one day, so you'll do what you can today, and then keep tackling it day by day and step by step, without attaching worry or anxiety.

→ **Let It Go[20]:** Here's how we're going to tackle this. I'm going to give you a list of things that you need to start letting go of. In turn, you will take that list and jot down an idea for each thing that you can start eliminating from your life.

Let go of...

- o Perfectionism
- o Comparison
- o People Pleasing
- o Regret
- o Guilt
- o Making Excuses
- o Blame
- o Fear of the Unknown

Here's an example from my journal:

Comparison - I see so many people on social media whose lives I wish mine looked like, I have to remember that I'm only seeing 2% of what their life is actually like. There's more behind the scenes than we realize - this also makes me want to gravitate more towards the people who are "keeping it real"...

That's a good place to start. The truth is there are likely 63 other things you could let go of, but I'm all about our motto here - **Keep It Simple**. These ones are the big ones - if you can tackle letting go of some of these weights that sit on your shoulders, you'll be well on your way.

"These mountains that you are carrying,
you were only supposed to climb."
~ *Najwa Zebian* ~

"Be here now" is my simple daily reminder to live in this moment, rather than the past or future. It helps me remember that I'm responsible for living my life to the fullest, not the life that comes from comparison to other people. It also grounds me in doing one focused thing at any given time, rather than becoming consumed by the hustle and bustle of juggling seven

---

[20] I know 50% of you sang that...

balls at once. A year into practicing this, it still doesn't come naturally. I seriously need a screensaver on my phone to remind me every single day, but I'm getting better at it and that's all the matters.

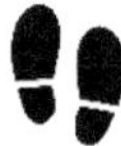 Your Next Steps:

→ **Practice Mindful Breathing:** Stop once a day (twice a day if you feel like a real go-getter) and breathe. But try to follow a sequence like this:
- Breathe in for the count of 3
- Hold for the count of 3
- Breathe out for the count of 3
- Repeat for 5-10 cycles

This exercise is a quick antidote to the tailspin of worry or hustle that you might find yourself in. Then remind yourself Be Here Now. And take a step to live in the present moment without worrying about yesterday of tomorrow.

"Be where you are. Otherwise you will miss your life."
~ Buddha ~

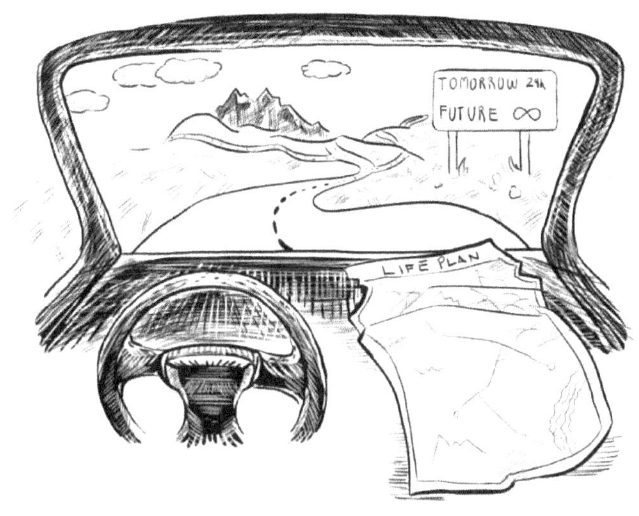

Get in the Driver's Seat

"Most people spend more time planning
a one-week vacation than
they spend planning their life."
~ Michael Hyatt ~

When I first read that quote by Michael Hyatt, I almost choked on my coffee.

It hit so close to home. I'm a vacation planner extraordinaire. I have spreadsheets, checklists, and detailed plans for every adventure we take. And why? Because I want our trips to go as smoothly as possible. I want us to get the absolute most out of our time away, a perfect blend of adventure with relaxation time weaved deliberately throughout.

Shouldn't I want the same from my life? One that flows as smoothly as possible, with goals being met and dreams becoming reality?

As I began living my life according to my motto "Be Here Now", I realized that I was getting better at intentionally living my life day-by-day. What about thinking forward to the future and using my day-by-day skills to build my months and years into exactly what I wanted them to be? I had a vision of what I wanted my life and our family's future to look like, and now making that vision become a reality was my main goal. I just needed a kick in the pants.

"I didn't come this far, to only come this far."
~ Unknown ~

Last spring I was at my annual visit with my gastro-enterologist - my specialist for all of my digestive issues. The receptionist checked me in and turned to get my chart from the shelf, "Woah, that's some file!" she commented as she plunked the stacks of folders and papers on the desk. As I took in both her comment and the monstrous size of paperwork from all the tests, procedures, and surgeries from the past 12 years, my heart filled with pride and a major sense of accomplishment. "I have come a long way..." I said to myself. Then as I sat in the room waiting for my doctor, I spent some time aimlessly scrolling through social media and a quote jumped out at me.

It said: "I didn't come this far, to only come this far." Those few words resonated deep down in my soul. I have overcome some major obstacles and the reality is that my ostomy surgery gave me a second chance at life. I would not let that life be wasted. And from that day forward, I've been attacking my dreams and goals with more drive and passion than ever before.

I truly believe that we all have obstacles and struggles that we've overcome. Taking a second to reflect on those can really help you gain motivation to move from the passenger's seat to the driver's seat.

Not sure which seat you're sitting in right now? Life in the passenger's seat looks like this:

- o Dreams floating around in your head but never becoming reality - *"I'd love to write a book one day..."*
- o Wishes for how you'd like your life to look - *"I wish we could go on a family vacation."*
- o Using the word "should" far too frequently - *"I should start exercising.", "I should start saving more."*
- o Always wanting to be better at something - *"I want to be a better mom.", "I want our marriage to be stronger.", "I want to take better pictures."*

Life in the driver's seat looks more like this:

- o Having goals written down with an action plan on how you're going to achieve them.
- o Consistently contributing to a savings account to help fulfil your wishes and dreams.
- o Understanding the power of the phrase "I will" and notice when you're making excuses with the phrase "I should".
- o Choosing an area of your life you want to improve in, by taking a course, reading a book, or finding a mentor to help you grow and succeed.

"If it is important to you, you will find a way.
If not, you will find an excuse."
~ Ryan Blair ~

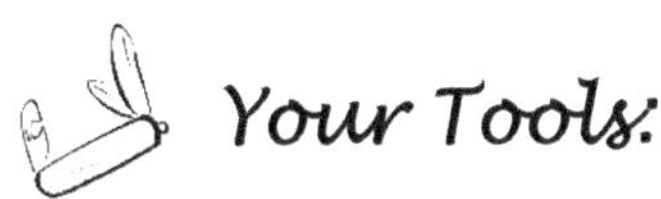 **Your Tools:**

→ **Eliminate the 'Luck' Roadblock:** If you continue believing that some people "are just lucky", you won't get very far. Your neighbour didn't get that promotion because he's lucky, and luck has nothing to do with your cousin being able to travel around the world. Taking action is the driving force behind most of the things we label as "luck". It really is that simple - take action.

→ **Identify Your Dreams & Goals:** Some of these sit up front and center and you know exactly what they are. Others are lying more dormant in the background, but they're just as important. Do another brain dump, listing all of the dreams and wishes you have, and labelling all of the goals that have been on your mind. Don't forget bucket list items on this list also. Maybe something like "meet the Queen of England" feels too far out of reach, but if it's something taking up space in your mind, it needs to come out on paper.

→ **Make Them Visual:** From your list, highlight your top 5-10. The ones that will make the biggest difference in your life right now. Now we get to revert back to our collage-making junior high selves and create a vision board.
  o Option One: Cut out pictures and words from magazines that reflect those dreams and goals and paste them on a piece of cardboard or pin them to a bulletin board
  o Option Two: Using an online collage making tool, like Canva or PicMonkey, take images and quotes you find online to create a vision board that you can print off and save as an image on the computer. I've done this and used it as my desktop wallpaper to keep it front and center.

Many people skip over this step, discounting its importance. Studies have proven that people who write down their goals and revisit them regularly are 50% more likely to achieve them. Look at this vision board every single day.

→ **Goal Setting:** You'll hear a lot of experts recommend setting five to ten goals per year. I personally believe that this is daunting so I set 90-day goals instead of year-long goals, and I pick one or two. For the moment - to see how successful you can become with driving your life forward - pick a single goal and write it out on paper. Under the goal, jot down things you would need to do to achieve it. After looking at that list of steps you need to take, decide which one needs to come first. What is one thing that you can do today to move you closer to your end goal? Now complete that step. Tomorrow when you wake up, look at your goal and decide what the *next* step is that you can do to move you closer to your end goal. Then do it. Put that simple cycle on repeat and you will achieve every single goal you set your mind to.

"Nothing happens until something moves."
~ *Albert Einstein* ~

The geek in me needed a mix of Albert Einstein and Isaac Newton to give me my final push. The law of inertia states that an object at rest stays at rest, and an object in motion stays in motion, unless acted upon by an external force. I just needed to stay in motion by taking another action step, every single day. My weight loss goal gained momentum by deciding every morning what physical activity I was going to add to my schedule. My vacation savings goal kept moving forward by waking up every day and deciding to not spend money on things we didn't need. Every goal moves forward when you decide on doing the next right thing.

 **Inspired By...**

Michael Hyatt & Daniel Harkavey: These two accomplished

and talented gentlemen wrote a book together called Living Forward. This book changed the way I think of goals and future planning. I moved from the passenger's seat to the driver's seat with their guidance and the exercises I completed in this book.

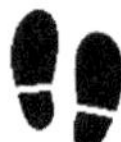 ## Your Next Steps:

→ **Start with your Goals & Dreams Brain Dump:** Spend some time on this, there is no need to rush it. Think deep and stretch your imagination.

→ **Then pick your top goal:** Choose one that will make the biggest difference in your life. Which one will help you become the best version of yourself? Chances are it's a personal goal and not a family vacation goal. Start there and have faith that you'll get to that vacation goal one day soon!

"You have brains in your head. You have feet in your shoes.
You can steer yourself any direction you choose."
~ *Dr. Seuss* ~

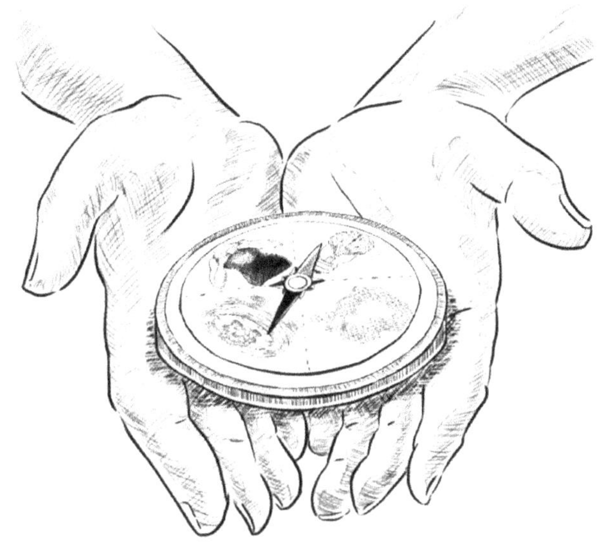

Grow Your Give Muscle

"Character is how you treat those
who can do nothing for you."
~ Unknown ~

Have you ever helped someone out who was in dire need, and felt that surge of happiness and pride inside afterwards? What a beautiful thing - that giving to others, actually gives back to yourself as well.

There is no better way to gain a sense of purpose and fulfilment in your life than to spend some of your time giving to a cause that you connect with. Your spiritual health will flourish when you feel like you are helping the greater good, fulfilling the lives of others and yourself at the same time.

There is no doubt that giving, in any way that you can, forever changes lives. That's such a powerful thought - to know that you have the ability to contribute to the world and in doing so, leave it a little better than you found it.

Strangely, there's a bit of an addictive nature to the act of volunteering - at least there has been for me. I have a tendency to get involved with too many causes and organizations, and eventually have to dial it back to a healthy amount that I can manage. Studies actually show that giving your time volunteering can raise dopamine levels in your body, giving you the same kick of pleasure that you get from eating a chocolate bar.[21]

"We make a living by what we get,
but we make a life by what we give."
~ Winston Churchill ~

My favourite part about volunteering for something near and dear to my heart is that it makes every single part of me feel good. What starts as healing my soul quickly spills over into every other area of my Compass.

My heart overflows as I connect emotionally to the people that I'm helping. When I work with a volunteer group, I connect with the others in that group as well. Those bonds are unique because they're rooted in working together towards the same

---

[21] Next advertisement campaign: "Volunteering – it's like eating a chocolate bar..."

greater purpose. These connections and bonds naturally decrease feelings of loneliness and depression.

My mind grows and develops as I build new skills in the particular area that I'm volunteering in. Those skills spill over into other areas of my life and I become more confident and motivated to continue helping others.

This ripple effect extends to my body as I feel less stress. Volunteering has proven to have positive physical side effects such as lower blood pressure. Amazing, right?

Above all, my soul experiences significant healing. When we can help bring life and meaning to whatever cause we're supporting, that purpose and meaning spreads to our own life as well. We can positively change ourselves by changing the lives of others.

"Volunteering is the ultimate exercise in democracy.
You vote in elections once a year, but when you volunteer,
you vote everyday about the kind
of community you want to live in."
~ Marjorie Moore ~

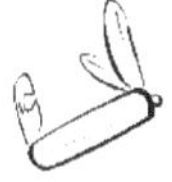 ## Your Tools:

→ **Identify What Matters To You:** This is different for everyone and it's important to realize that. Just because your best friend loves giving her time to the SPCA, doesn't mean that you have to. Think about what is important to you and make a short list of causes you would give your time or money to.

  o **Find Your Cause:** This might be easy as you may already know exactly where you want to volunteer. However if you don't, here are some places to start your search:
  In Canada:

- o **Volunteer Canada - www.volunteer.ca -** a site dedicated to "increase the participation, quality and diversity of volunteer experiences".
- o Search regionally or locally based on your province and town/city, by simply typing in "volunteer _____" into good ol' Google.

In the United States:
- o **Volunteer Match - www.volunteermatch.org -** they want to help you find a cause that "lights you up".
- o **Idealist - www.idealist.org -** is an organization dedicated to moving you from intention to action. They believe that too many good ideas go unheard and strive to match you with a cause that really matters.

→ **Realize that Time > Money:** Although it's true that every single organization can use the gift of donation money to help their cause, you should remember that it helps even more when you volunteer your time. Donations are important and shouldn't be forgotten, if you have the means to contribute. But place a greater value on donating your time – that's what both your soul and your cause needs.

"Only by giving are you able to receive
More than you already have."
~ Jim Rohn ~

Dedicate some time to find a volunteer opportunity that speaks loudly to you. What are you passionate about? The world needs you and your passions - let's give to help ourselves heal and to change the world around us.

 **Inspired By...**

Altruistic Current: "Reflect the world you want to see". Their vision is simple, to promote altruism - intentional acts of kindness towards any living beings without the expectation of reciprocation - within our communities. They believe that altruism is for everyone and that we can change the world, one person, one community, and one city at a time. Their projects are amazing. All pay-it-forward in nature, and every time that I watch one of their events unfold on social media my heart grows ten-fold just being a passive participant.

Timber Coffee Company (Sylvan Lake, AB): More than half of the DNA of this book was born out of this fabulous café. The atmosphere is always a perfect blend of background noise, but also quiet enough to focus. Their lattes are, bar none, the best I have tasted in visiting coffee shops on three different continents. Their staff are the kindest people in the world. But the best thing ever – they are a non-profit organization with proceeds given to local youth programs. I love spending my money in places that benefit the community as a whole.

Kindness Matters: - John Magee of the Kindness Matters movement in the UK, spreads his message daily by sharing random acts of kindness everywhere he goes. He has a very engaged and active community on Facebook and his Instagram feed and stories are among my favourite to follow. He says, "Kindness very rarely costs a thing, but the value is priceless." I couldn't agree more. The most simple of things - a smile or holding the door open for someone - can have such a huge impact in the lives of others. He has a 30-day Kindness Challenge which encourages people to complete one Random Act of Kindness every single day and journal about what you did and how it felt. I personally love that every day on Instagram, John shares a Kindness Tip - something quick and easy that we can incorporate into our lives, to spread kindness into the world around us.

👣 *Your Next Steps:*

→ **Discover your cause:** Dig deeper into discovering what's important to you and search out the organization that you can start donating your time with. Reach out to them and ask what you can do to help.

→ **Bonus Points:** Start with a simple smile. When you're out in public, smile often at the people you meet along the way. It can make a big difference in someone's day, and is the easiest gift you can give.

"At the end of the day it's not about what you have or even what you've accomplished. It's about who you've lifted up. Who you've made better. It's about what you've given back."
~ *Denzel Washington* ~

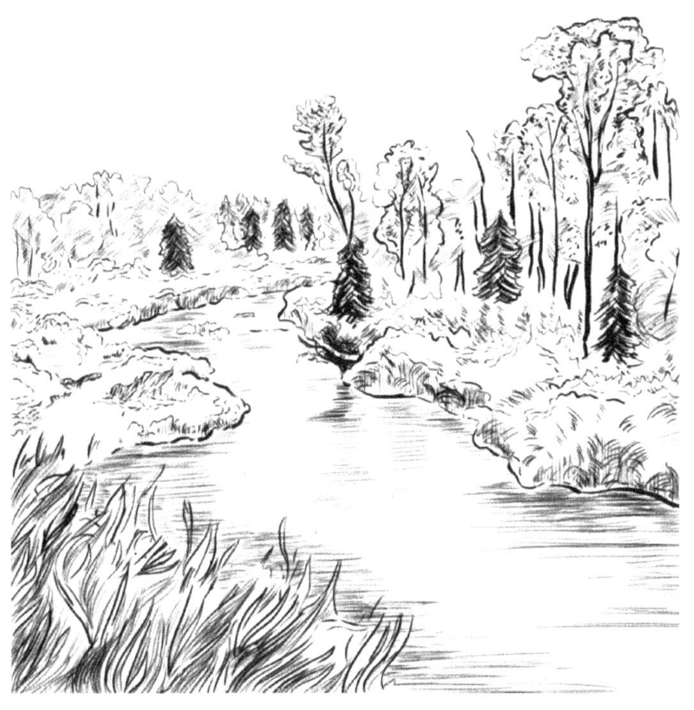

Back to Nature

"The earth plays music for
those who listen."
~ *William Shakespeare* ~

When I was a kid, I was immersed in the natural world around me. Rolling in the grass, playing in the mud, and running through the trees - these activities just came naturally, my parents didn't have to teach me how to do them. I think most people can relate. As a kid you spend hours lost in fresh air and the smells of trees, fresh cut grass, and mud puddles.

Then we get older. And for many of us, we become far removed from those basic back-to-nature pastimes. It makes me sad to think that I'll likely spend more of my life staring at a computer screen than staring at the trees. So, I try to make it my mission to get outside and experience everything glorious that Mother Nature has to offer.

There's a poetic side to being in nature. Like the undeniable fact that your heart is softened, your mind slows down, and your soul opens up, whenever you spend time with the ocean, trees, lakes, mountains, or rivers.

"To walk in nature is to witness a thousand miracles."
~ Mary Davis ~

There is science behind the healing powers of nature. Anything that blends science with poetry is the most beautiful thing in my eyes. Here's why you need to spend more time in nature:

→ **Vitamin D** - The only place you can naturally get this vitamin is from the sun. You can take supplements, but they are no replacement for actually getting sunshine on your body. There have been studies linking the lack of Vitamin D to certain inflammatory and autoimmune diseases like mine, so this is a **big** one in my book. You need to be exposing your skin to sunlight regularly, and in every season, even when you live in places where snow falls over six months of the year.

→ **Better Sleep** - Your body's sleep pattern works with

something called the circadian rhythm, an internal clock that helps regulate when you fall asleep and when you wake up. This rhythm works best when it's naturally tied to the sun's schedule. However when you spend most of your time indoors, away from natural sunlight and exposed to lots of artificial light, your circadian rhythm gets disrupted and consequently your sleep can suffer. Studies have shown that getting back outside, exposing yourself to natural light and fresh air, can get that rhythm and your sleep back on track.

→ **Healing Your Body -** Most likely, getting outside will lead to exercise, even in the form of a gentle walk. It's hard to have one without the other - when you're in nature, you move. Movement and exercise has huge benefits on your overall health: lower rates of depression and anxiety, increased mental clarity, and a better functioning immune system. Get outside and move. Treadmills have their benefits for sure, but a walk outside does your body a world of good.

→ **Less Stress -** An impressive "nature therapy" study, conducted in Japan, tested 420 subjects in 35 different forests throughout the country. They removed the subjects from their primarily urbanized lives and tested various physiological functions during their time in nature. They found a decrease in heart rate, as well as lower levels of cortisol (the stress hormone) when compared to subjects who remained in the city. Their findings suggested that nature therapy should play an increasingly important role in the future of preventative medicine.

Nature heals us - Body, Mind, Heart, and Soul - there's no denying it. But like most things that we know are good for us, we don't need to be convinced of *that.* We just need to know how to make it happen in our lives. We need the tools to make sure our souls see more of Mother Nature than of Google.

---

*"Wisdom comes with the ability to be still.
Just look and just listen. No more is needed."*
~ Eckhart Tolle ~

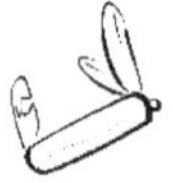 *Your Tools:*

→ **Camping and Hiking:** It helps that two of my absolute favourite hobbies involve being out in nature for long stretches of time. Our family gets out on a handful of camping trips every summer and there is absolutely nothing like being in the middle of nowhere surrounded by nature. That's right, we don't camp in campgrounds - we head out to the wide open spaces where there are no hookups, no amenities, and plenty of quiet. Try one or both of these activities if they're not something you already do.

→ **Letting the Kids Choose:** Spend some time connecting to kids, whether they're yours, nieces or nephews, or other kids you know. Take them to a park or playground, or even better, for a walk in nature. Let them lead and you'll be amazed at what they teach you. Like how to slow down, how to appreciate the little things, and how to unwind, laugh, and just be.

→ **Make Dates with Mother Earth:** One of the indigenous names for Mother Earth is Pachamama. I think that's a beautiful name. So you'll actually see this in my personal calendar on a weekly basis: "Date with Pachamama". At least I try my hardest to put it in there every week. These dates are chunks of time where I try to get at the very minimum 15 minutes, but more likely 30-60 minutes of time spent outside. This varies on the season - winter often sees weeks at a time where we're stuck indoors because the temperature dips to -30°C. But in the spring/summer/fall, I make time for a short walk or even eating lunch outside in the grass - this makes a huge difference to my spiritual health. Try making your own dates with Mother Nature.

"I took a walk in the woods, and came out taller than the trees."
~ Henry David Thoreau ~

Your soul will become replenished and open up in such a beautiful way when you can slow down and find stillness in nature. When you find that place of stillness, your vision becomes clearer and you can finally hear what your heart has been whispering all along.

 **Inspired By...**

Melissa Hartwig – I first mentioned this mentor back in the Body section and the benefits of her Whole 30 program. She's inspired me in my spiritual healing as well. I follow her personal Instagram account where she shares pictures of the various hikes she does in the beautiful mountains of Utah. She talks about how being in nature and surrounded by beauty is where she feels the most intense spiritual connection of all - she calls it her church. And I totally agree - being in nature, finding stillness, and seeking quiet - that's where my church exists too.

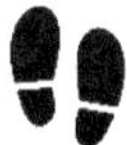 # Your Next Steps:

→ **Put it in your calendar:** Make your first date with nature. Find a chunk of time this week that you can get outside for a short and simple walk. If you're in the city, try and make the walk happen in a nearby park so that you can be closer to the grass and trees and further from the cement and skyscrapers.

→ **Step outside for ten deep breaths of air:** Sometimes making an actual date with nature is difficult due to weather, the season, or illness. In this case, try stepping out your front door at least once a day to breathe ten deep breaths of fresh air. It'll make a difference, I promise.

"Because sometimes lying under trees and walking barefoot on the Earth is the most spiritual thing you could ever do in your life."
~ Unknown ~

Your Compass

Are you ready to become a mapmaker? You've become more familiar with all of the tools and have a clear understanding of how our Body, Mind, Heart, and Soul are all interconnected. Some of the chapters likely spoke loudly to you, while others you filed away into the "not-my-thing" drawer.

I'll share a secret that I've learned about that "not-my-thing" drawer. It's often full of the things that we might need the most in our lives. Sometimes it's fear of the unknown or a closed mindset that causes us to file things away in that drawer. If you choose to tell yourself "I'm open to trying new things" and give something an honest try, you may be surprised by the things that make the biggest difference in your life.

Let's go over the two parts of the system. You have your Compass, which you will use at the beginning of each month to assess how you're feeling in each area – your Body, Mind, Heart, and Soul. Then you have your Tracker, which you will use every day to both remind yourself and track your progress of the healthy habits you are using to help heal.

Visit **www.myhealingcompass.com/compass** to print a copy of your Compass and Tracker (in colour). It will look like this:

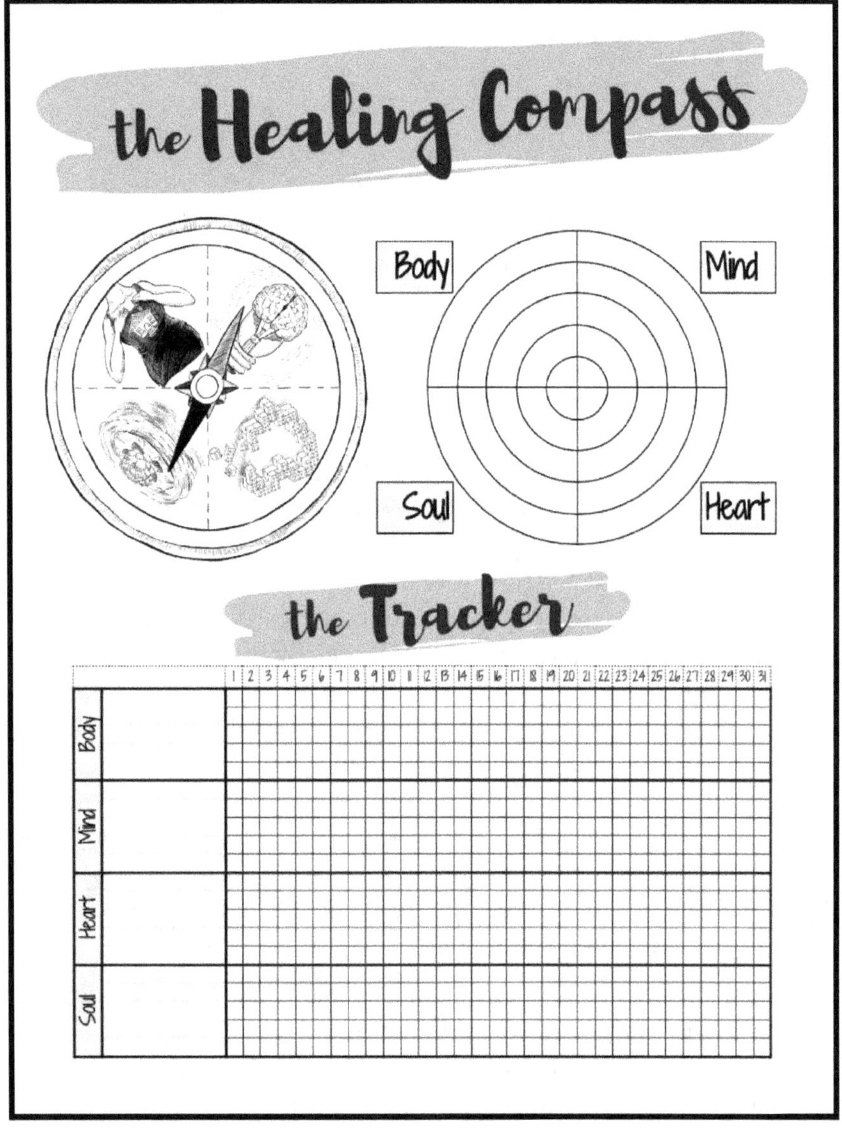

In the top right-hand corner of the page, you will see your Compass. This is where you assess the four areas of your health at the beginning of each month. On a scale of 1-5 (one being the worst and 5 being the best), how do you honestly feel in each area? Remember, your areas are:

Body = Physical Health
Mind = Intellectual Health
Heart = Emotional Health
Soul = Spiritual Health

Questions to ask yourself would be things like:

Body (Physical Health)	Mind (Intellectual Health)
o How does my body feel? Achy-breaky? Or full of energy? o What have I been putting in my body? Nutritious foods or mostly junk? o Have I been active lately? Or more sedentary?	o Does my mind feel clear or foggy? o Have I been pushing myself to learn something new? o Does my life feel organized or chaotic?
Soul (Spiritual Health)	Heart (Emotional Health)
o Can I sit in quiet and feel peace inside of me? Or unrest? o Do I have current goals written down? o Have I been worrying about the future, or fretting about the past?	o Am I reacting quickly to triggers? Or pausing to respond? o Do I feel connected or disconnected to family and friends? o Have I been taking care of Me?

After filling it out, your Compass may look like this:

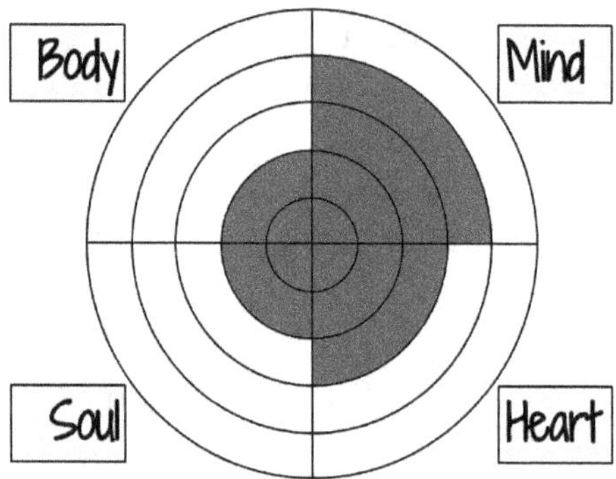

This can change substantially in just one month's time, depending on where you intentionally put your focus every day. By first recognizing which part of yourself needs a little more attention, you can add in some simple steps to help that area heal. As time goes on, it becomes easier as certain habits become more natural.

Your next step is to look at your Tracker and decide which habits you're going to work on this month. Remember, these aren't meant to be earth-shattering changes. They are small, simple steps you can easily accomplish to start living a healthier, happier life. Let's take a look at that tracker:

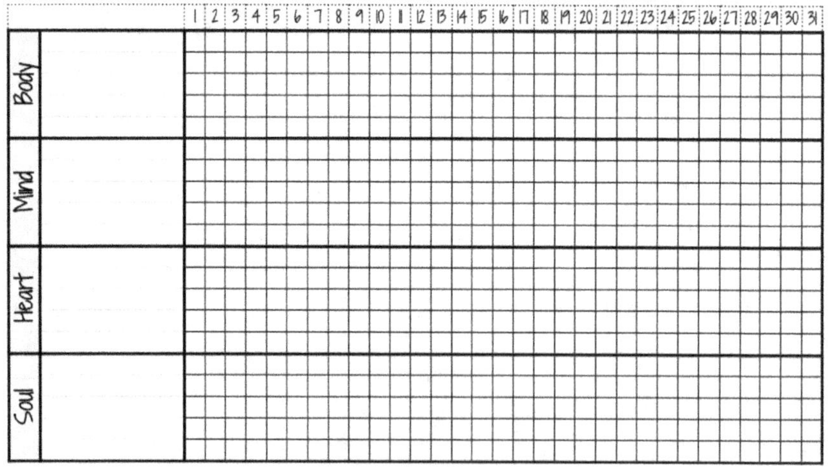

In the beginning, choose just one or two habits for each area of the Compass. It really does depend on where you're at in your journey. Look at the Compass that you just filled out as your monthly check-in. Which area(s) need the most love and attention right now? Focus here first.

Next, move on to the other areas of the Compass that are either mediocre or you're doing great with. Choose one or two habits for these areas as well. I like to include a balance of habits I'm currently doing with habits that aren't part of my regular routine, to see which ones will help make a difference.

Here is a reminder of the chapters we've covered, plus a list of potential habits you could start tracking. Remember, the goal is not to "do it all". Pick one or two in each area that make sense for **you**.

Body	
Let's Get Moving	Exercise, Walk, Yoga, Stretch, Move
Eat Like Great-Grandma	Track meals, No sugar, Eat at home, More veggies
Catch Those Zzzz's	Go to bed on time, No screen in bed, 7-8 hours sleep
Tune Into Your Body	Body scan, Jot journal, Pause during day
Build Your Health Posse	Make appt., Visit healer, Home exercises (for physio, etc.)

Mind	
Your Brain Needs Fuel Too	Read for fun, Read for growth, Puzzles, Practice language
The Stress of Stuff	Declutter, File, Tidy up, Brain dump, Fill up donation box
Boss of the Clock	Planning time, Less social media, Focused work

Find Your Drumbeat	Me time, Win the day, House time, Meal planning
Do What You Love	(Insert hobby here...)

Heart	
Medicine for Your Heart	Timeout when upset, Honour losses, Let something go
Pen & Paper	Gratitude journal, Line-a-day journal, Write letter
Connect The Dots	Connect with spouse, Connect with kids, Connect with friend
A New Kind of Self-Care	Food for body, Food for mind, Food for heart, Food for soul
Finding Dandelions	Sit with pain, Journal hurt feelings, Choose joy

Soul	
Can You Hear That?	Meditate, pray, sit in silence
Be Here Now	Mindful breathing, Slow down, Let it go (one thing)
Get in the Driver's Seat	Check in with goals, Look at vision board
Grow Your Give Muscle	Volunteer, Save for donations, Collect for food bank
Back to Nature	Step outside, Go for walk, Breathe fresh air

Now, put it to practice.

- o **Step One:** Wake up in the morning and take a look at your Tracker. Where are you going to fit these habits into your day? Are there any that you can do right now to have an immediate win and check the box?
- o **Step Two:** Review your Tracker again at the end of the day. Is there anything you can do now to help you keep moving in the right direction (for example, going to bed on time)? Is there anything you can put into your calendar tomorrow to make sure it happens?
- o **Repeat. Every single day.**

Okay, this next part is important. And it's coming straight from the mouth of a recovering perfectionist. Your Tracker will never look perfect. There will always be off days. It will likely resemble something like this:

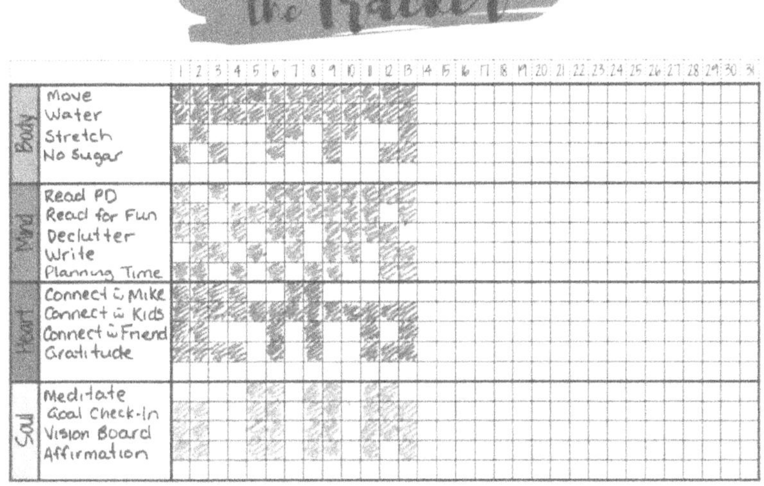

Focus on progress, not perfection. That example above is me having a really good month. There were a couple of things that I focused on every day, with no excuses. For this particular month I added more movement and connected with my kids each day. As for everything else, they remained in my general focus area way more than before I started using this system, but I don't worry or stress about having an off day. Life happens. We just don't want it to steamroll us.

Zero stress and no worries are the name of the game. Start singing Hakuna Matata at any time. So, as you start using your Compass and Tracker, it will be natural to have those moments and days where you start to feel overwhelmed or frustrated that you're not seeing progress, or that you completely forgot about the entire thing for a whole week.

Pause. Take a step back, and possibly remove one or two things from your Tracker and start tomorrow with a fresh perspective and a deep breath.

Your Healing Compass isn't going anywhere. The more committed and intentional you are in making the necessary changes or shifts in your life, the better you'll feel and the more healed you will become.

This journey is worth it. Trust me. You can do this, step by step, and day by day. Remember: **Keep it Simple.** You can find your unique roadmap to the healthiest and happiest version of yourself. Just by taking care of yourself, and feeling the connection between your Body, Mind, Heart, and Soul every single day.

Remember, life has a way of getting away from us. Our days will blend into weeks, months, and then years without us making any progress towards our goals and the life of our dreams. So don't wait until tomorrow. There is no one more important than yourself. Start the journey today. I'm here for you every step of the way.

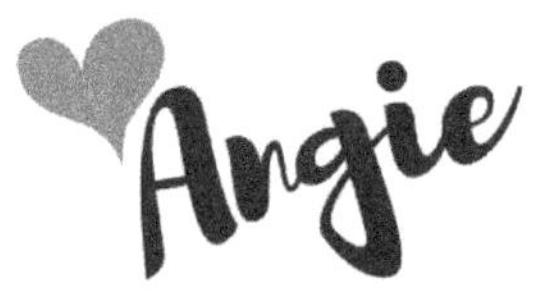

Acknowledgements

Every time that I've sat down to write this page - the one that thanks the many beautiful souls that have helped me get here - I end up in a puddle on the couch, snuggled up with my favourite blanket.

I've been warned that I have a tendency to over-exaggerate and that I love hyperbole a little bit too much... but everything I'm about to say cannot be said without lots of "amazing's", "best-ever's", and "with all of my heart". Forgive me for using overzealous hand gestures and repeating the "I love you's" 27 times. This is a section of the book that my editor wasn't allowed to touch. Ha ha, surprise Erin! (So please forgive me for any and all grammatical errors. I'm shooting straight from the hip here.)

This may sound ridiculous to some, but I have actually spent sleepless nights with my monkey mind worrying that I'm over my quota of amazing people in my life. Seriously. As if I'm walking up to Border Customs and I'm going to be forced to declare myself over the limit of awesome friends and family. And you know those bastards are going to tax me on that over-the-limit-of-awesomeness. Right?

 Every single one of you better know who you are already, because I have made it a life goal to never let my feelings go unknown. I try to express my gratitude and love unabashedly, from the rooftops (except I'm scared of heights so it's more like "from the step-stool"). But in case I've been slacking in my expression of love and gratitude lately, forgive me and let me declare it all over again.

Let's make this fun. Pour yourself a glass of wine, crack a beer, craft a cocktail, brew some tea or coffee, or grab your water bottle (you know, in case you're doing some crazy elimination reset like I suggested back in the Body Section). Raise your glass with me for every "Cheers" just to honour all of these amazing souls. (I think that's only two "amazing's" - I'm doing pretty good so far...)

First of all, Cheers to everyone who is reading this - Thank you for being my readers, whether you are new-found or old-school friends. Thank you for letting me hand over a piece of my heart and soul, entrusting you not to stomp on it. And thank you for that too - for taking my words and giving them a home in your homes, and for not sending me hate mail. One of my biggest fears is hate mail. Can you believe that I almost didn't follow my dream of writing a book, merely for fear of one person hating it? Haters gonna hate. (Thanks Taylor). I've gotten over it.

Cheers to all of My Newfound Cheerleaders - You know who you are. I've met you in coffee shops, my husband has chatted your ear off on an airplane, or we met on the beaches of Cuba. All of you newfound acquaintances who quickly became friends, thank you so much for your support and encouragement. To have strangers listen to my story and my dream, and watch them scrawl their email address on the nearest cocktail napkin, has made my heart grow ten-fold. (Who am I kidding? That's my sucker for romance side showing - realistically they sent me a text so that I had their number. Do cocktail napkins even exist anymore?). Thank you newfound friends and cheerleaders for giving me a bigger trampoline to jump off of towards my dreams.

Cheers to My Small Town Family. There is this amazing thing that happens when you grow up in a rural community. You automatically inherit a dozen sets of parents, grandparents, aunts, uncles, and cousins. Your graduating class of 24 remain your close friends for life even when you scatter your separate ways, always standing in your corner whether you're suffering from loss or pursuing your dreams. My original small town has 1000 people and my current small town has 150. I'm afraid I'll go over my page limit if I list ALL of you - but you know who you are. I know that you do, and I thank you with all of my heart.

Cheers to My People that I found after leaving the safe bubble of a small town. I have to share a really quick anecdote from moving into residence in the big city, my first year of university. My mom and sister moved me into my dorm and my roommate (who had already clothed our small room in black Curt Kobain flags on the windows and walls), introduced herself as "Hi, I'm Sarah. I don't like people". My shy, timid self wanted to cry and beg my Mommy not to leave, but instead this crazy roommate pairing forced me to get out of my room more and meet some of the most amazing people in the world. Leslee, Shireen, Michelle, Camille, Mya, Steph, Heather (and honestly every other res friend I made) - thank you for sticking with me through some of the craziest and most memorable years of my life. And thank you for being there still today.

Cheers to the Best Friends I could have ever asked for - The ones who send cards or flowers "just because". The ones who drive two hours out of their way for a "quick visit". The ones who know exactly what I need before I even know it myself. The ones who meet me for playdates and both of us have Mommy Brains so our conversations barely make sense but we can finish each other's sentences so it doesn't even matter. The ones who have sent me the most encouragement, the most love, and the most support over the last 20 years. Brandy, Kelly, Shireen & Les - your love is buried so deep in my heart. Trac – thank you for being my rock and for wading through so much of the deep with me. My piano toes still play every morning for you. And Jen - thank you for helping me grow, for kicking my butt when I need it, and for loving my hubby and kids with all of your heart. And thank you to your hubby and kids for being the best cheerleaders ever. We've seen so many dark days and so many happy endings together - that kind of friendship has healed me in a way that you totally get, because I know you feel it too.

Cheers to my "other families" – I worked as a nanny for ten years, both part-time and full-time for three of the most amazing families ever. Duncan & Melinda, Rick & Christine, Eggy & David – I hope you know that your families have left an everlasting imprint on my heart. The support and unconditional love you have given me over the years has been incredible, and your kids will always be remembered as "my kids" for the brief periods of time that I was lucky enough to be their nanny. Ethan, Emily, Mia, Anna, Ethan & Henry (yes, there was two Ethan's) – oh my gosh, we have shared so many fun memories together. All of you will always have the uncanny ability to put the biggest smile ever on my face.

Cheers to the Best In-Laws Ever - Wanna know who gets super excited about their mother-in-law coming for a visit? This girl. I married into such an amazing family - Stephanie, Roy, Uncle Mike, Chris, Becki, Cassie, and Kayleigh - your love and support since the day that I walked into your family, is so very much appreciated. "Grandma-Who-Brings-Us-Candy" - I love having a second Mom who loves me like I was her own daughter. "Grandpa-On-The-Farm" - I love our visits, and I love still having a dad to come and visit after I lost my own. Audrey - I miss you more than I could ever put into words. You witnessed so many of my sickest days, and our chats made a world of difference during that time. I miss your listening ear and beautiful smile.

Cheers to the Biggest Family in the World - Between my Dad's 11 brothers and sisters and all of their children, grand-children, and great-grand-children; plus my Mom's 8 brothers and sisters and all of their children, grand-children, and great-grand-children; not to mention extended family, third cousins twice removed... you get the picture. I not only have the biggest family in the world, but pretty much the best. And I'm thankful that the internet has made our world that much smaller so that we can keep in touch so much easier.

Cheers to My Brudder & Seesters, and their families. Randy - I know that my five year old self used to drive your 17 year old self bonkers, but thank you for playing Go Fish with me anyways, and in general putting up with me. I love that we have grown so close over the past ten years. Pam – I love the feeling of having someone who "just knows". Thank you for being someone to look up to, someone to listen to my triumphs and my woes, someone to laugh with over the silly things, and someone who has been by my side through some of the hardest days of our lives. Vicki - your spirit has been cheering me on from the day this book idea started becoming a reality. Losing you has left this gaping hole in our lives, but in that hole I found the seeds for becoming my whole self again, and I'm reminded that on the other side of darkness there will always be light. I know how much you loved peace and quiet, so you're probably getting tired of me constantly talking your spiritual ear off, but thank you for listening. I feel you around me constantly.

Cheers to the rest of our humungous family – Marcia, Mel, Jim, Lynds, Tyler, Sam, Andrew, Amber, Dylan, Jas, Skylar, Dan, Dayton, Dustin, Jordan, Matt, Jared, Ashley, Quinn, Holly, Jason, Shawna, Landon, Brooke, Josh, Kandi, Dominic, Emryck, Rylan, Gracie, Hannah, Emma, Nolan, Baby-on-the-way. Phew, that's just the immediate family. I love having special, totally unique, relationships with each and every one of you. When you think of the quilt or puzzle our family creates, blended together, it's a masterpiece for sure. Omg – that's like 34 cheers in one fell swoop. This wasn't supposed to be a drinking game.

This book didn't get here on its own. Who else fell in love with the drawings in each chapter? There were days where those illustrations were the only thing that kept me going because I was like, "they can't live in this world without a story attached to them!" Here I go, all cliché on you (my editor would've definitely nixed this...) – "A picture is worth a thousand words..." – but seriously, I wanted to include images in this book that would reflect the ideas that have become so important and influential in my life. My illustrator Amber Solberg went above and beyond with every single image. She knew what my heart conveyed even when I couldn't find the exact words. She took super vague ideas of mine ("a heart that has feelings") and made them a reality. Cheers to you Amber.

Cheers to my editor – Erin Dyrland. I think being an editor is similar to being a wedding photographer or wedding planner. The Author-zilla side of things isn't pretty. I only had a handful of those panicked "this is all going to hell in a handbasket!" moments. But thank goodness Erin answered all of my crazy phone calls, emails, and texts to help me get back to "cool cucumber" status. I hated every second of the editing process even though I love the finished product one hundred times more than my first chicken scratches that only made sense inside my head. Erin, thank you for being so patient and kind and telling me my thoughts made zero sense when you needed to. I also loved the hugs, hand drawn hearts on pages, and high fives. And thank you for always having the answer to every problem (real or imagined) that I ~~was freaking out about~~ shared. Oh, and the Oxford Comma – thank you for that.

Now, this is where I get really weepy. I've used a handful of tissues already. Hand over the whole box...

Cheers to my mom and dad - you planted every single seed that has made me the person I am today. And more than that, you nurtured those seeds with so much love, encouragement, pride, and support. I seriously can't find the words to express my gratitude for every little and big thing you have done for me over the years. Mom - you've been my biggest confidant since day one, and throughout every stage of life that felt uncertain and confusing you've kept squeezing my hand to remind me that everything is going to be okay. You gave me that first push to become an author. Do you remember "The Muppets Save Christmas?" Dad - I miss you with every fiber of my being. I miss your gentle smile, your desire to argue politics and climate change with me, and your love of everything that brought me joy. I miss your voice on the phone. I miss you being my lifeline during Trivial Pursuit with Mom. I miss the hours we spent together watching hockey, shooting hoops, playing chess, beating each other at Jeopardy, and laughing at the Royal Canadian Air Farce.

To my beautiful babies - everything that I do, I do for you. Thank you for being my greatest teachers and for the zillions of smiles, laughs and huggles that you've brought into our lives. Cassie, Lincoln and Savannah - you are the sunshine in my life every single day. I love you with all of my heart, and I am so grateful to be in this place of healing so that I can soak up every second that I have with you.

My Mike - I will be grateful for eternity that you came over and started chatting with me that fateful February night that feels like forever ago. You have been the person my soul needed to help me grow into the best version of myself. Your support and cheerleading throughout this book-writing journey has helped ground me and let me fly, all at the same time. There is no one in the world that I'd rather share this crazy adventure with. Here's to growing old and grey together, traveling the world, and me always laughing at your corniest of jokes. I love you.

"The secret to having it all, is knowing you already do."

Notes

Your Body:
Melissa & Dallas Hartwig, *The Whole 30: The 30-Day Guide to Total Health and Food Freedom.* (Toronto: Penguin Group, 2015) **www.whole30.com**

Let's Get Moving:
Daniel & Kelli Segars, *Fitness Blender,* **www.fitnessblender.com**

Adriene Mishler, *Yoga with Adriene,* **www.yogawithadriene.com**

Rubin, Gretchen, *Better than Before: What I Learned About Making and Breaking Habits – To Sleep More, Quit Sugar, Procrastinate Less, and Generally Build a Happier Life,* (pg 211), (Anchor Canada: 2015)

Sandi-Rae Hebb, *Peace in a Pod Yoga Studio,* **www.peaceinapodyoga.com**

Eat Like Great Grandma:
Rory Hornstein, RD., *RoryRD.com,* **www.roryrd.com**

Lisa Leake, *100 Days of Real Food,* **www.100daysofrealfood.com**
Cookbooks:
   100 Days of Real Food: How We Did It, What We Learned, and 100 Easy, Wholesome Recipes Your Family Will Love. (New York: Harper Collins, 2014)
   100 Days of Real Food: Fast & Fabulous: The Easy and Delicious Way to Cut Out Processed Food. (New York: Harper Collins, 2016)

Danielle Walker, *Against All Grain,* **www.againstallgrain.com**
Cookbooks:
    Against All Grain: Delectable Paleo Recipes to Eat Well and Feel Great. (Las Vegas : Victory Belt Publishing, 2013)
    Danielle Walker's Against All Grain: Meals Made Simple: Gluten-Free, Dairy-Free, and Paleo Recipes to Make Anytime. (Victory Belt Publishing, 2014)
    Danielle Walker's Against All Grain Celebrations: A Year of Gluten-Free, Dairy-Free, and Paleo Recipes for Every Occasion. (Berkeley: Ten Speed Press, 2016)

Catch Those Zzzz's:
Arianna Huffington, *The Sleep Revolution: Transforming Your Life, One Night at a Time,* (Harmony Publishing, 2016)

National Sleep Foundation, *"What Happens When You Sleep",* (no date) **www.sleepfoundation.org/how-sleep-works/what-happens-when-you-sleep**

Build Your Health Posse:

Emma Loewe, *"Reiki: What It Is + Why You Should Consider Adding It to Your Routine"*[online article]. Available: **www.mindbodygreen.com/0-23414/reiki-what-it-is-why-you-should-consider-adding-it-to-your-routine.html** (October 20, 2017)

Your Mind:
Greg McKeown, *Essentialism: The Disciplined Pursuit of Less.* (New York: Crown Business, 2014)

Your Brain Needs Fuel Too:
Ann M. Martin, *The Baby-Sitters Club Series,* (Scholastic, 1986)

J.K. Rowling, *The Harry Potter Series,* (London: Bloomsbury Publishing, 2000)

Andrew Merle, *"The Reading Habits of Ultra-Successful People"* [online article]. Available: **www.huffingtonpost.com/andrew-merle/the-reading-habits-of-ult_b_968813** (November 21, 2017)

Sadie Trombetta, *"Why Reading is the Best Workout for your Brain"*[online article]. Available: **www.bustle.com/p/why-reading-is-the-best-workout-for-your-brain-57441** (November 3, 2017)

Website: Good Reads (**www.goodreads.com**)

Anne Bogel, *Modern Mrs. Darcy,* **www.modernmrsdarcy.com**

Lewis Howes, *School of Greatness Podcast,* **www.lewishowes.com/blog**

Gretchen Rubin & Elizabeth Kraft, *Happier Podcast,* **www.gretchenrubin.com/podcasts**

Tsh Oxenreider et. al, *The Simple Show Podcast,* **www.theartofsimple.net/thesimpleshow**

Jenna Kutcher, *Goal Digger Podcast,* **www.podcast.jennakutcher.com/**

Emily P. Freeman, *The Next Right Thing,* **www.emilypfreeman.com/podcast/**

The Stress of Stuff:
Gretchen Rubin, *"Fighting Clutter: Go Shelf by Shelf",* [online article]. Available: **www.gretchenrubin.com/2011/02/fighting-c**

Tsh Oxenreider, *The Art of Simple,* **www.theartofsimple.net**

Marie Kondo, *The Life-Changing Magic of Tidying Up: The Japanese Art of Decluttering and Organizing,* (Berkeley: Ten Speed Press, 2011)

Boss of the Clock:
David Allen, *Getting Things Done: The Art of Stress-Free Productivity,* (New York: Penguin Books, 2015)

Find Your Drumbeat:
Rubin, Gretchen, *Better than Before: What I Learned About Making and Breaking Habits – To Sleep More, Quit Sugar, Procrastinate Less, and Generally Build a Happier Life,* (pg 211), (Anchor Canada: 2015)

Crystal Paine, *The Money Saving Mom,* **www.moneysavingmom.com**

Kendra Adachi, *The Lazy Genius Collective,* **www.thelazygeniuscollective.com**

Do What You Love:
Mark Manson, *"Screw Finding Your Passion",* [online article]. Available: **www.markmanson.net/passion**

Paula Timm, *Paula Timm Artist Studio,* **www.paulatimm.com**

Pen and Paper:
Cathy Malchiodi, *"Creativity as a Wellness Practice",* [online article]. Available: **www.psychologytoday.com/blog/arts-and-health/201512/creativity-wellness-practice**

Brené Brown, *The Gifts of Imperfection: Let Go of Who You Think You're Supposed to Be and Embrace Who You Are,* (Minnesota: Hazelden Publishing, 2010)

Brené Brown, *Daring Greatly: How the Courage to be Vulnerable Transforms the Way We Live, Love, Parent, and Lead,* (New York: Penguin Random House, 2012)

Brené Brown, *Braving the Wilderness: The Quest for True Belonging and the Courage to Stand Alone,* (New York: Random

House, 2017)

A New Kind of Self-Care:
Shauna Niequist, *Present Over Perfect: Leaving Perfect for a Simpler, More Soulful Way of Living,* (Grand Rapids: Zondervan, 2016)

Hal Elrod, *The Miracle Morning: The Not-So-Obvious Secret Guaranteed to Transform Your Life (Before 8AM),* (Hal Elrod, 2012)

Your Soul:
Thompson River's University, *"Spiritual Wellness",* [online article]. Available: **www.tru.ca/wellness/my-wellness/spiritual.html**

Can You Hear That:
Andy Puddicombe & Rich Pierson, *Headspace,* **www.headspace.com**

Michael Acton Smith & Alex Tew, *Calm,* **www.calm.com**

Kris Carr, *Self-Care for Busy People,* **www.kriscarr.com/buy-selfcare-meditationalbum**

Get in the Driver's Seat:
Michael Hyatt & Daniel Harkavey, *Living Forward: A Proven Plan to Stop Drifting and Get the Life You Want,* (Grand Rapids: Baker Books, 2016)

Grow Your Give Muscle:
Altruistic Current, **www.altruisticcurrent.com**

Timber Coffee Co., **www.facebook.com/timbercoffeeco**

John Magee, *Kindness Matters,* (John Magee, 2017)

Back to Nature:

Lauren F. Friedman & Kevin Loria, *"11 scientific reasons you should be spending more time outside"* [online article]. Available: **www.businessinsider.com/scientific-benefits-of-nature-outdoors-2016-4/#1-improved-short-term-memory-1** (November 12, 2017)

Your Compass:

Elton John & Tim Rice, *Hakuna Matata,* (Disney, The Lion King, 1994)

Acknowledgements:

Taylor Swift, *"Shake It Off",* (Big Machine Records, 2014)

Coming Soon...

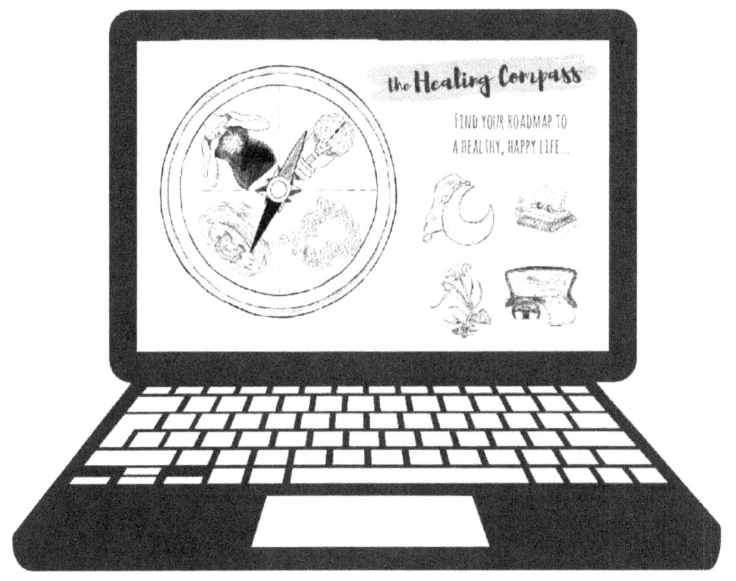

the Healing Compass E-course & Online Workshops

TAKE A DEEP DIVE INTO HEALING YOUR BODY, MIND, HEART & SOUL
THROUGH AN ONLINE COURSE WITH PERSONAL COACHING!

Sign up at www.myhealingcompass.com for more details!